PASSING
CALCULATIONS
TESTS in NURSING

PASSING [4TH EDITION]
CALCULATIONS
TESTS in NURSING

SUSAN STARKINGS & LARRY KRAUSE

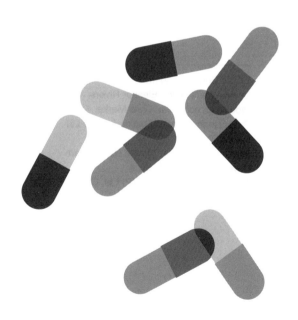

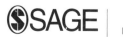SAGE | LearningMatters

Foreword for the third edition

Nurses are expected to have many different skills; in one minute they are practising the art of emotionally supporting and caring for a patient in distress and in the next they turn to science and mathematical skills to calculate medications. Numeracy is one of those essential ingredients in a nurse's repertoire of skills and this text concentrates on honing the skills nurses need in the basic medicines calculations that are required to assist in the care and treatment of their patients.

You will find in this text extremely clear and easy-to-follow instructions to revise, or learn from scratch, the methods you will need to calculate medications and work out metric conversions, fluid balance and intravenous infusions. There is a self-test to guide your learning and a final chapter that helps you prepare for tests and examinations. The text itself is a tonic to take away the panic of drug calculations!

The authors, Susan Starkings and Larry Krause, will provide you with scenarios and case studies to help give context to the situations you will encounter in drugs calculations. It will not give you, however, the detailed pharmacological knowledge or rationales for treating with medications or calculating volumes and quantities. This knowledge is also a fundamental ingredient of managing the care of patients. For this you will need to read further texts in the series on medicines managements; this will provide you with that essential underpinning knowledge to enable you to integrate mathematics with your therapeutic role in care.

The authors have provided a wealth of extra questions and material on the online resources. The online questions provide an opportunity for extra practice and self-testing so you can monitor your progress and check that you have understood the techniques introduced in the book.

I know you will gain confidence and competence from reading and working through the superbly well-written exercises in this text. Good luck with your examinations and your improved numeracy skills, which will add another feature to your growing portfolio of practice skills.

Shirley Bach
Series Editor

Acknowledgements

The publisher and authors would like to thank Heather Short, RGN, Dip/DN, BSc (Hons), MEd, Senior Lecturer, University of the West of England, Bristol, and Patrick Saintas, Principal Lecturer, Faculty of Health and Social Sciences, School of Nursing and Midwifery, University of Brighton, for their helpful comments on early drafts of the first edition of this book.

How to use the online resources

The online resources that accompany this book provide students with ready-to-use activities to help with everyday studies and revision. They are free of charge and are designed to maximise the learning experience.

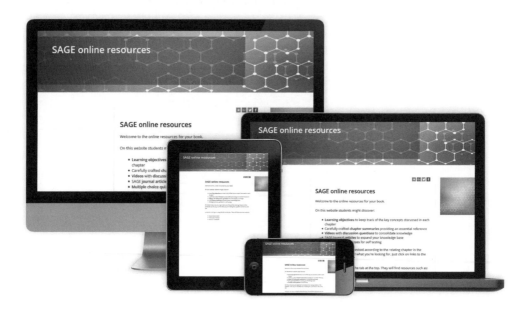

You can access the website via your computer, laptop, tablet or smart phone at **https://study.sagepub.com/starkingskrause4e**

On the website you'll find …

- **Online self-tests and extra questions.** When it comes to success with calculations, the key is practice, practice, practice. To help with this the authors have provided a bank of over 400 extra questions available on the website.

- **Interactive glossary.** To help you learn or revise key terms introduced in the book, try out the flashcard glossary.

- **Useful websites.** There is a huge amount of helpful information available on the internet that will help you to improve your mathematics and numeracy skills and the authors have provided a range of recommendations for you.

Introduction

The aim of this book is to put the calculations required for nursing into the practical contexts that you should encounter during your training. It was written after seeing, over many years, the problems that student nurses commonly encounter. The text aims to address these problems using realistic examples.

Book structure

The book has been designed to supplement your nursing studies and to be used for self-study. The first chapter contains a diagnostic test. We suggest that you try out this test first to identify which areas of numeracy you need help with. Then work through the chapters relevant to the area(s) identified; when you feel that you have understood these areas, re-do the diagnostic test and compare the results from your first attempt. Chapter 2 contains the basic arithmetic required for nursing calculations. Chapter 3 shows you how to convert from one metric quantity to another, and Fluid Balance Charts are covered in Chapter 4. A simple and effective method to calculate the correct drug dosage in liquid, tablet or capsule form is in Chapter 5. How to calculate the required rate of an intravenous drip rate using the most commonly found equipment values is covered in Chapter 6, while calculating children's drug doses is covered in Chapter 7.

Finally, Chapter 8 will help you prepare for any calculations tests you might be taking, and includes advice on how to prepare for the test, revision questions and tips on common errors to avoid.

Learning features

Each chapter begins with an outline of what is covered in the chapter. The chapter content has been written to help you meet the requirements of the Nursing and Midwifery Council (NMC) *Standards for Pre-registration Nursing Education* (NMC, 2010) and Essential Skills Clusters (ESCs) as well as the *Standards of Proficiency for Registered Nurses* (NMC, 2018). These are a set of requirements about what skills and competencies you will need to demonstrate in order to become a registered nurse; your nursing programme will have been designed around them. The NMC were undertaking a revision to these nursing skills and competencies at the time of writing and so the authors have kept the existing NMC requirements and incorporated the draft NMC requirements into this fourth edition. There are specific requirements for medicines calculations and numeracy that you should be aware of and work towards. These are included here (from both sets of standards) for your reference.

NMC Standards for Pre-registration Nursing Education 2010

27(2) Accurately monitors dietary and fluid intake and completes relevant documentation.

28(1) Takes and records accurate measurements of weight, height/length, body mass index and other appropriate measures of nutritional status.

29(2) Accurately monitors and records fluid intake and output.

33(1) Is competent in basic medicine calculations.

32(2) Monitors and assesses people receiving intravenous fluids.

33(2) Is competent in the process of medication-related calculation in nursing field.

36(4) Safely manages drug administration and monitors effects.

38(4) Safely and effectively administers and, where necessary, prepares medicines via routes and methods commonly used and maintains accurate records.

NMC Essential Skills Clusters

- Numeracy skills.
- Drug calculations required to administer medicines safely via appropriate routes including specific requirements for children and other groups.

NMC Standards of Proficiency for Registered Nurses 2018

1.13 Demonstrate the literacy, digital literacy, technological literacy and numeracy skills required to ensure their safe and effective nursing practice.

4.11 Demonstrate the principles of safe and effective optimisation and administration of medicines in accordance with local and national policies. Demonstrate proficiency and accuracy when calculating dosages of prescribed medicines (Annexe B).

Annexe B:

- undertake accurate drug calculations for a range of medications including insulin and controlled drugs;

- record fluid intake and output and identify signs of dehydration or fluid retention;
- accurately measure weight and height, calculate body mass index and recognise healthy range and clinical significance of low/high readings.

An additional possible draft requirement for the new standards is for Continuing Professional Development (CPD) and a potential requirement of 3 Year Re-Registration within the Profession with some testing to obtain/retain qualifications.

The authors have therefore included in Chapter 8 a small series of tests for those looking to undertake CPD to achieve Non-Medical Prescribing (NMP) Nurse qualifications; for these nurses more examples will also be placed on the book's accompanying website. Should there ever be a requirement for nurses to re-register by the NMC or regulatory authorities then this edition, along with the website's online questions, should assist in those studies/re-registration and with your CPD.

Case studies and scenarios are introduced throughout the text to illustrate the relevant nursing calculations, and each chapter has activities, with solutions, for you to try.

There is a glossary of terms at the end of the book that provides an interpretation of some of the terminology in the context of the subject of the book. Glossary terms are in **bold** in the first instance they appear.

This book does not cover all nursing calculations, and questions, scenarios and case studies are as realistic as possible but are not related to any real person. To obtain maximum benefit from this book, it is suggested that you work through the diagnostic test in Chapter 1 first.

A note on terminology

Please note that it is recommended that micrograms and nanograms should not be abbreviated in practice – that is, using the symbols 'mcg' and 'ng' (*British National Formulary* (BNF) (2014) *BNF* 68. London: BMJ Group/Pharmaceutical Press). Abbreviated forms of measurements have been used occasionally in this book to save space. Great care should be taken not to confuse mg (milligrams) with mcg (micrograms) and ng (nanograms) as this can lead to errors. However, there may be occasions when you see these abbreviations in books, journal articles or even on patients' prescriptions. You must always follow your Trust/employer and university policies regarding the approved abbreviations that you are allowed to use.

Chapter 1 Diagnostic assessment

Chapter aims

By the end of this chapter you will have:

- completed the diagnostic test;
- identified areas of numeracy that you need help with from your diagnostic test results;
- selected the relevant chapter(s) that would be useful to aid your studies.

Introduction

Nurses need to achieve competence in numeracy skills in order to cope safely with calculations. These skills are essential to the safe administration of medications and general nursing calculations involved with patient care for both adults and children. Nurses do not need higher degree qualifications in mathematics, so do not worry. Essential nursing calculations will be covered in this text to help you achieve the skills required for safe nursing practice.

Calculator usage

Most nursing calculations carried out for assessment purposes are usually performed without the use of a calculator so it is important that you can do the calculations manually (on paper) or in your head. It is therefore recommended that the questions in the chapters are answered without the use of a calculator. You can, should you wish, use a calculator to check your answers for the purpose of studying, but carry out the calculations manually first.

Diagnostic test

The purpose of this exercise is to highlight the numeracy and mathematics required for the modern nurse. Attempt the diagnostic test, without using a calculator, to assess your current understanding and mathematical ability. Solutions are provided at the end of this chapter, along with advice on which chapters within this book to refer to for further assistance or revision. Appropriate online resources that you could use to aid your learning further, and for practice purposes, are recommended. The two main websites that have been recommended here are BBC Bitesize and the Higher Education Academy Centre for Excellence in Teaching and Learning Mathcentre website. You may also like to use the Open University (OU) OpenLearn website, which gives free access to learning materials.

For this test you do not need any prior knowledge of healthcare or nursing terminology. The aim of the test is for you to ascertain your own numerical and mathematical ability in addition, subtraction, multiplication, division, fractions, decimals, percentages, ratios, factors and metric conversions, all of which will be used throughout your future career as a registered nurse.

This diagnostic test is designed to allow you to determine your current level of mathematical ability; it is not a speed test. Hence you may take as long as you feel necessary to undertake this exercise. It is suggested that you complete the test by yourself to ascertain your own strengths and weaknesses in your numerical and mathematical ability. Seeking assistance at this point will not give you a true indication of your strengths and the areas in need of further revision.

Each section, consisting of ten questions, introduces you, the future registered nurse, to some of the calculations needed to accurately determine the correct amount of medication to be given to your future patients. In later chapters you will use the skills tested here to carry out the more specialised nursing calculations you will use throughout your career.

The questions below cover the maths you need to accurately complete the range of nursing calculations covered in this book as well as those you will see as a registered nurse. At the end of the test, check your answers and make an assessment of where you need to start. Alternatively, you can work through the whole book and come back to the diagnostic test at a later stage.

There is no need for you to worry if you cannot do some of the questions at this stage, since you can work through the book at your own pace to improve your numerical and mathematical ability.

It is your decision what chapter or chapters you wish to work through once you have identified gaps in your skills from your results in the diagnostic test. If you wish to know your percentage score for the test, just add up the number of questions you answered correctly; this number is also the percentage score that you have obtained (because there are 100 questions).

Now work through each section and identify what chapter you need to start with. Work at your own pace, and remember that it is not a speed test.

Addition and subtraction

Calculate the following:

1. $1600 + 750 =$
2. $150 + 36 =$
3. $2750 - 527 =$
4. $1441 - 1326 =$
5. $1500 + 35 - 16 =$
6. $(129 - 42 + 95) - (79 + 13) =$
7. $(68 + 35) - (21 - 17) =$
8. $321 + 169 - 27 =$
9. $29 + 714 - 592 =$
10. $(820 - 123) + (550 - 218) =$

Addition and subtraction are among the basic numeracy skills essential for nursing calculations, so it is important for you to be able to do these accurately. Should you have any difficulty with addition and subtraction, it is suggested that you start at Chapter 2 (Essential numeracy requirements for nursing) and work your way through this book. You may also like to use the online BBC Bitesize practice material. This website has examples and practice questions for you to try out and check against the solutions. For addition and subtraction, use web pages 1 and 2 listed at the end of this chapter.

These numerical calculations are required for many areas of nursing, especially **Fluid Balance Charts**; see Chapter 4 for examples, scenarios and case studies.

Multiplication and division

Calculate the following:

11. 279×1000
12. 320×2.75
13. $275 \div 25$
14. $27.5 \div 2.5$
15. $1043 \div 7$
16. 0.321×1000
17. 0.079×1000
18. 9.214×100
19. $342.8 \div 10$
20. $72.98 \div 100$

Should you have any difficulty with multiplication and division, it is suggested that you start at Chapter 2 and work your way through this book. You may also like to use web pages 5 and 6 listed at the end of this chapter.

Multiplication and division are used extensively for the quantity conversions covered in Chapter 3, and in the drug calculations that you will see in Chapter 5. For example, you will need to be able to convert milligrams to micrograms and centimetres to millimetres as part of your routine tasks.

Fractions

Write the following in their simplest form:

21. $\dfrac{5}{20}$

22. $\dfrac{50}{100}$

23. $\dfrac{50}{150}$

24. $\dfrac{49}{105}$

25. $\dfrac{125}{450}$

26. $\dfrac{34}{136}$

27. $\dfrac{275}{1000}$

28. $\dfrac{52}{6}$

29. $\dfrac{132}{5}$

30. $\dfrac{29}{9}$

For drug calculations, the simplification of fractions is an essential skill. Should you have any difficulty with questions 21–30, it is suggested that you start at Chapter 2. For online practice, use web pages 3 and 16 (BBC Bitesize) listed at the end of this chapter.

Multiplying and dividing fractions

Solve each of the following, leaving your answer as a fraction in its lowest terms:

31. $\dfrac{25}{125} \times \dfrac{10}{1}$

32. $\dfrac{1}{4} \times \dfrac{8}{15}$

33. $\dfrac{4}{5} \times \dfrac{5}{1}$

34. $\dfrac{1}{2} \div \dfrac{2}{3}$

35. $\dfrac{6}{7} \times \dfrac{14}{60}$

36. $\dfrac{13}{30} \div \dfrac{26}{90}$

37. $\dfrac{2}{3} \div \dfrac{6}{5}$

38. $\dfrac{25}{125} \div \dfrac{10}{1}$

39. $\dfrac{5}{9} \div \dfrac{36}{15}$

40. $\dfrac{3}{5} \times \dfrac{1}{5}$

Most of the drug calculations you will be required to perform use these types of calculations. If you have any problems here, start at Chapter 2. For online practice, use web page 4 (BBC Bitesize); for the rules of arithmetic, see web page 18 (Mathcentre) listed at the end of this chapter.

In Chapter 5 you will find examples of drug calculations requiring these types of numerical skills. Children's nursing also requires these skills, and Chapter 7 has examples of child nursing calculations that all nurses, not just children's nurses, should be familiar with.

Decimals and percentages

Write the following as fractions in their simplest form:

41. 0.75	46. 1.5%
42. 0.375	47. 0.02
43. 20%	48. 15%
44. 0.05	49. 12%
45. 75%	50. 0.525

A drug concentration can be given in the form of a percentage of the total volume available; hence you need to be able to interpret percentages and convert them to fractions in order to calculate the dosage required for your patient. Throughout Chapter 5 (Drug calculations) you will meet examples using this type of numeracy. For example, if you have to dilute a solution, say to clean a wound, then you will need to understand percentages. Fractions and decimals will be covered in Chapter 2; if you find these practice questions difficult, start at this chapter. For online practice you could use web pages 8 and 10 (BBC Bitesize) or 15 and 17 (BBC) listed at the end of this chapter.

Fractions and percentages

Convert each of the following to a decimal:

51. $\dfrac{1}{5}$	56. 41%
52. 10%	57. $\dfrac{25}{100}$
53. $\dfrac{1}{8}$	58. $\dfrac{1}{20}$
54. 35%	59. 9%
55. $\dfrac{5}{10}$	60. 20%

It is essential that you can convert between fractions, percentages and decimals easily and quickly. Decimals will be covered in Chapter 2; if you find these questions difficult, it is advised that you start at this chapter. Downloadable booklets on fractions, decimals and percentages can be found on web pages 15, 16 and 17 (BBC); web page 10 (BBC Bitesize) is also a good online resource with which to supplement your study.

Units of measurement

Find the equivalent metric measure for each of the following. The use of the unit of measure is a critical part of the answer.

61. 0.75g = ? mg
62. 10mg = ? micrograms
63. 320ml = ? litres
64. 725g = ? kg
65. 20 microgram = ? nanogram

66. ? g = 2500mg
67. ? kg = 1500g
68. ? litres = 2100ml
69. ? mg = 75g
70. 1.5 mole = ? millimole

Please see note on page 3 concerning the use of abbreviations.

Questions 61–70 test your knowledge of the units generally used in clinical medicine and by nurses in the giving of medications. It is vital that you can accurately convert from one unit to another; this is required for many of the drug calculations that you will carry out as part of your duties as a registered nurse.

Conversion from one unit to another is one of the most common sources of error in nursing. This can be dangerous: an overdose could lead to further health complications or prove fatal, while an underdose may impede a patient's recovery as the medication may not function correctly. Chapter 3 (Quantity conversions for nurses) covers the conversions most commonly used in nursing calculations; if you made any errors in the above questions, Chapter 3 would make an ideal starting point. For online practice, see web page 14 (BBC Bitesize).

Other calculations involving conversions include the calculation of intravenous (IV) drip rates; in Chapter 6, for example, a conversion from hours to minutes is used. For online practice with units of time, see web page 7 (BBC Bitesize) listed at the end of this chapter. However, before attempting Chapter 6, make sure you have covered and understood the processes and procedures covered in Chapter 3.

Ratios and factors

Convert the following ratios to percentages:

71. 1 in 10
72. 1:49
73. 1 in 20
74. 1 in 50
75. 1:24

Work out the following factors:

76. Which of the numbers 2, 3, 5, 7, 9 are factors of 128?
77. What are the prime factors of 65?
78. The prime factors of 15 are ...?
79. What is the common prime factor of 25 and 35?
80. What is the common prime factor of 69 and 48?

You need to understand the ways in which the strength or dilution of a solution is written on the labels of any medication that you deal with in practice. Liquid solutions may be labelled with a ratio (or proportion of volume): for example, '1:1000 adrenaline' is a typical format that you might see on the hospital ward. Chapter 2 explains the use of ratios; for online practice, see web page 11 (BBC Bitesize); for practical examples of ratios, see Chapter 5 (Drug calculations) and Chapter 6 (Calculating intravenous rates).

It is beneficial to know what the factors of numbers are because this makes cancelling down, which is used in drug dosage calculations, easier. Familiarisation with factors will improve your speed at all types of nursing calculations, especially when working without a calculator, as is required for your formal assessments. Most of the formal assessments you have to do as part of your training will be timed and hence a certain amount of speed is required. For online practice in number factors, see web page 12 (BBC Bitesize).

Rounding decimals

Round the following to one decimal place:

81. 39.1367	86. 725.08
82. 1.86	87. 4.92
83. 600.652	88. 0.7216
84. 2000.29	89. 0.1952
85. 43.36	90. 0.15

Some of the nursing calculations you do will not give a whole number answer, and you will need to round the answer to an appropriate degree of accuracy: to a whole number or to a certain number of decimal places. Rounding of numbers will be covered in Chapter 2; online practice can be found on web pages 13 (BBC Bitesize) and 19 and 20 (OpenLearn).

The final ten questions in this diagnostic test are 'word questions'; they are closer in style and type to the nursing calculations you will have to do during your training. In case study tests, a scenario will be given in a written format and it is the student's or trainee's task to understand and obtain all the relevant information required to calculate the answer; case studies are presented throughout this book so that you can practise these skills. Some trainee nurses find this style easier as the questions are more realistic; however, the numeracy required to undertake them is similar to the previous questions in this test.

Word questions

The use of the unit of measure is a critical part of the answer.

91. Write the following number in figures: two thousand, three hundred and sixty-four.
92. How much is 20% of 600g?
93. What is two litres in millilitres?
94. In a ward of 20 patients, four of them are under two years of age. What percentage of these patients is over two years old?
95. Complete: 25 gram = ? milligram
96. How many minutes are there in two and a quarter hours?
97. Mr Blake is ordered 20mg of phenobarbitone to be taken orally. Tablets in your medicine cabinet are 10mg tablets. How many tablets does Mr Blake need?
98. Mrs Bush should have a **fluid intake** of two and a half litres. She has drunk the following: 500ml of coffee twice, 250ml of tea, 200ml of orange juice and 500ml of water. How much more fluid should Mrs Bush take to reach the two and a half litres required?
99. Miss Rebecca Grant must have nil by mouth for 8 hours before her operation, which is scheduled for 7 a.m. At what time must you start her nil by mouth? (Answer in 24-hour time format.)
100. Mr Hume was given 50ml of water per hour for 8 hours. How many millilitres in total did he receive?

If you find these ten questions difficult, re-read them and pick out the relevant information required for the calculations. For online help with units of time, see web page 7 (BBC Bitesize) listed at the end of this chapter.

Hint ... There are lots of context-based questions throughout this book to give you the practice you need. Read on and spend some time on the areas that you have identified as problematic. Read the chapters you have identified as most relevant and work through the scenarios, case studies and practice questions included.

If you have had few problems with the above questions, you might prefer to start at Chapter 4 and work your way through the following chapters in order to make sure you can do the nursing calculations covered accurately. You can always refer back to an earlier chapter should you need to refresh your memory on any aspect of numeracy. Chapter 2 covers the basic numeracy required to start your nursing calculations.

Useful websites

BBC Bitesize

The BBC Bitesize online resources offer revision material that you can use to enhance your numeracy and mathematical skills. The web pages below have been referenced in this chapter and are accessible free of charge.

1. Addition

    www.bbc.co.uk/schools/ks2bitesize/maths/number/addition/read1.shtml

2. Subtraction

    www.bbc.co.uk/schools/ks2bitesize/maths/number/subtraction/read1.shtml

3. Cancelling fractions

    www.bbc.co.uk/schools/gcsebitesize/maths/number/fractionsrev3.shtml

4. Multiplying and dividing fractions

    www.bbc.co.uk/schools/gcsebitesize/maths/number/fractionsrev22.shtml

5. Long multiplication

    www.bbc.co.uk/schools/gcsebitesize/maths/number/multiplicationdivision rev1.shtml

6. Long division

    www.bbc.co.uk/schools/gcsebitesize/maths/number/multiplicationdivision rev2.shtml

7. Units of time

    www.bbc.co.uk/education/topics/zj48q6f

8. Decimals

    www.bbc.co.uk/schools/gcsebitesize/maths/number/decimalsrev1.shtml

9. Percentages

   www.bbc.co.uk/schools/gcsebitesize/maths/number/percentagesrev1.shtml

10. Converting fractions and decimals

    www.bbc.co.uk/schools/gcsebitesize/maths/number/fracsdecpersrev1.shtml

11. Ratios

    www.bbc.co.uk/schools/gcsebitesize/maths/number/ratiosrev2.shtml

12. Prime factors

    www.bbc.co.uk/schools/gcsebitesize/maths/number/primefactorsrev1.shtml

13. Rounding decimals

    www.bbc.co.uk/schools/gcsebitesize/maths/number/roundestimaterev2.shtml

14. Converting measurements

    www.bbc.co.uk/schools/gcsebitesize/maths/shapes/measuresrev1.shtml

15. Decimals

    www.bbc.co.uk/education/topics/zh7xpv4

16. Fractions

    www.bbc.co.uk/education/topics/zsxhfg8

17. Percentages

    www.bbc.co.uk/education/topics/zf6pyrd

Mathcentre

Another useful free online resource is the Higher Education Academy Centre for Excellence in Teaching and Learning Mathcentre which offers students quick reference guides, practice and revision materials, video tutorials, workbooks and online practice exercises on many branches of mathematics. For nurses the following areas contain useful extra practice material and have been referenced in this chapter.

18. Rules of arithmetic

    www.mathcentre.ac.uk/students.php/health/arithmetic/rules/resources/

OpenLearn

The OU OpenLearn website gives free access to learning materials from higher education courses. The following pages are relevant to your nursing studies.

19. Numbers, units and arithmetic

    www.open.edu/openlearn/skills-for-study

20. Rounding and estimation

    www.open.edu/openlearn/skills-for-study

Visit the online resources on your computer at **https://study.sagepub.com/starking skrause4e** or on your smart phone or tablet and gain access to:

- over 400 extra questions to check your learning and gain extra practice;
- links to useful websites that build on the skills introduced in this chapter;
- an interactive glossary of key terms.

Answers to the diagnostics test

1. 2350
2. 186
3. 2223
4. 115

5. 1519
6. 90
7. 99
8. 463

9. 151
10. 1029

Your score:

If you scored seven or less you may wish to go to Chapter 2.

11. 279 000
12. 880
13. 11
14. 11

15. 149
16. 321
17. 79
18. 921.4

19. 34.28
20. 0.7298

Your score:

If you scored seven or less you may wish to go to Chapter 2.

21. $\frac{1}{4}$
22. $\frac{1}{2}$
23. $\frac{1}{3}$
24. $\frac{7}{15}$

25. $\frac{5}{18}$
26. $\frac{1}{4}$
27. $\frac{11}{40}$
28. $8\frac{2}{3}$

29. $26\frac{2}{5}$
30. $3\frac{2}{9}$

Your score:

If you scored seven or less you may wish to go to Chapter 2.

31. 2
32. $\frac{2}{15}$
33. 4
34. $\frac{3}{4}$

35. $\frac{1}{5}$
36. $\frac{3}{2}$ or $1\frac{1}{2}$
37. $\frac{5}{9}$
38. $\frac{1}{50}$

39. $\frac{25}{108}$
40. $\frac{3}{25}$

Your score:

If you scored seven or less you may wish to go to Chapter 2.

41. $\dfrac{3}{4}$

42. $\dfrac{3}{8}$

43. $\dfrac{1}{5}$

44. $\dfrac{1}{20}$

45. $\dfrac{3}{4}$

46. $\dfrac{3}{200}$

47. $\dfrac{1}{50}$

48. $\dfrac{3}{20}$

49. $\dfrac{3}{25}$

50. $\dfrac{21}{40}$

Your score:

If you scored seven or less you may wish to go to Chapter 2.

51. 0.2

52. 0.1

53. 0.125

54. 0.35

55. 0.5

56. 0.41

57. 0.25

58. 0.05

59. 0.09

60. 0.2

Your score:

If you scored seven or less you may wish to go to Chapter 2.

61. 750mg

62. 10 000mcg

63. 0.32l

64. 0.725kg

65. 20 000ng

66. 2.5g

67. 1.5kg

68. 2.1l

69. 75 000mg

70. 1500 millimole

Your score:

If you scored seven or less you may wish to go to Chapter 3.

71. 10%

72. 2%

73. 5%

74. 2%

75. 4%

76. 2

77. 5 and 13

78. 3 and 5

79. 5

80. 3

Your score:

If you scored seven or less you may wish to go to Chapter 3.

81. 39.1

82. 1.9

83. 600.7

84. 2000.3

85. 43.4

86. 725.1

87. 4.9

88. 0.7

89. 0.2

90. 0.2

Your score:

If you scored seven or less you may wish to go to Chapter 2.

91. 2364

92. 120g

93. 2000ml

94. 80%

95. 25 000mg

96. 135 minutes

97. 2 tablets

98. 550ml

99. 2300hrs using a 24-hour clock format

100. 400ml

Your score:

If you scored eight or less you may wish to go to Chapter 5.

Total score: number of questions you answered correctly = your percentage score.

Chapter 2 Essential numeracy requirements for nursing

Chapter aims

By the end of this chapter you should be able to:

- cancel down fractions;
- multiply decimal numbers by other decimal values;
- divide decimal numbers by other decimal values;
- convert fractions to decimals;
- convert decimals to fractions;
- round decimal and fraction values as appropriate;
- convert time fractions and decimals to minutes;
- carry out addition and subtraction.

Introduction

Patients and service users rely on nurses to accurately calculate and administer their medication. Too little could see the patient not recovering in the manner that would be expected; too much could have potentially harmful or fatal consequences.

The numeracy and calculations required of nurses are not difficult once practised and you will not need to use a calculator. Activities are included throughout this book for you to attempt without using a calculator. This chapter will lead you through the best-practice methods of determining the correct answers for all the calculations you will encounter as a successful nurse.

As a nurse you will carry out many calculations, ranging from dosage of medication for your patients to the hydration levels on their Fluid Balance Charts. The mathematics required is not difficult and with practice is readily mastered. If you are worried about the maths you need as a nurse, then you have the right book; throughout this chapter you will see the easiest way in which to overcome your fears of the mathematics needed to become successful. The skills you will learn in this chapter will be used in the other chapters of this book and will be invaluable throughout your nursing career. They will also enable you to pass your drugs calculation tests.

It may seem a challenge to you at the moment but with practice and determination you will become proficient in all elements of the mathematics used in nursing.

One of the first things required is a basic knowledge of multiplication tables. To some people this can be daunting. However, it need not be so as just four numbers are enough to start with. If you know the times tables for the first four **prime numbers**, you can 'cancel down' most numbers.

2   3   5   7

These numbers are the first four prime numbers, meaning they can be divided only by themselves and one. All other numbers can be built by multiplying combinations of prime numbers. Two of the prime numbers listed above are very powerful as they can be used to cancel down three out of every five numbers, no matter how many digits they have.

Hint ...

If a number ends in   0 or 2 or 4 or 6 or 8

Then it is divisible by 2

If a number ends in   0 or 5

Then it is divisible by 5

Cancelling down fractions

When cancelling down a fraction, the numbers on the top and bottom of the fraction must be cancelled by the same value at the same time. You do not have to use the same value each time you cancel and could use different values at different times. The numbers being divided must divide exactly by whatever value you are cancelling down with.

Hint ... When cancelling down a fraction, the numbers on the top and bottom of the fraction must be cancelled by the same value at the same time.

In Chapter 5 (Drug calculations) we look at liquid, tablet and capsule doses; the calculations involved are much simpler if you have cancelled down. For this worked example only part of a drug calculation will be shown.

Worked example

As part of a drug calculation you need to cancel down the following fraction.

$$\frac{225}{900}$$

The fraction ends in 5 on the top and 0 on the bottom, so both numbers are divisible by 5.

$$\frac{\cancel{225}}{\cancel{900}} = \frac{45}{180}$$

Again, the numbers on the top and bottom of the fraction can be divided by 5 as they end in 5 or 0.

$$\frac{\cancel{45}}{\cancel{180}} = \frac{9}{36}$$

Having cancelled down this far, it is still possible to divide top and bottom. This time you can divide by 3 twice or by 9 once (9 being 3×3) – these are the only number/s that both 9 and 36 can be divided by exactly.

$$\frac{9}{36} = \frac{3}{12} = \frac{1}{4}$$

This fraction, one-quarter, is the same as the original fraction and cannot be cancelled any further. It is much easier to use in nursing calculations than the original fraction.

In all the chapters of this book your ability to cancel down will be reviewed time and again; it is a core skill that you will require throughout your career.

In the above worked example, you may have noticed that you could have cancelled down using the factor 25 for the two first cancelling down actions. Provided you are comfortable working with a larger number like this, there is no reason not to do so. Given time, you may even build your confidence and ability levels sufficiently to use numbers like 125. For now, just be aware that $125 = 25 \times 5$, or $125 = 5 \times 5 \times 5$, and so dividing by 125 is the same as dividing by 5 three times in succession. Similarly, in Chapter 5 (Drug calculations) you will see that cancelling down by 16 is the same as dividing by 2 four times in succession, because $2 \times 2 \times 2 \times 2 = 16$. The importance of practice cannot be emphasised enough; the more you do, the better, faster and more accurate you will become at the numeracy skills required as a nurse.

Activity 2.1

Cancel down the following fractions to their simplest form, dividing top and bottom until no further number is exactly divisible into both parts of the fraction.

(Continued)

(Continued)

1. $\dfrac{675}{900}$ 2. $\dfrac{400}{850}$ 3. $\dfrac{5}{75}$ 4. $\dfrac{6}{104}$ 5. $\dfrac{17}{51}$ 6. $\dfrac{16}{96}$

7. $\dfrac{3}{75}$ 8. $\dfrac{75}{300}$ 9. $\dfrac{13}{104}$ 10. $\dfrac{96}{480}$ 11. $\dfrac{228}{528}$ 12. $\dfrac{35}{85}$

Answers to all the activities can be found at the end of the chapter.

Multiplying decimals

Some students become anxious when confronted with numbers containing a decimal point. Nurses need to be able to multiply and divide numbers with a decimal point in either one or both numbers. Just as with the cancelling of fractions, what you need is practice.

Case study

Brenda works in a mental health clinic where a service user, Ahmed Mustapha, has been prescribed 0.375 grams of venlafaxine daily. To ensure there is sufficient stock on hand she has been asked to calculate in grams the amount of venlafaxine required for Ahmed for a 7-day period.

Brenda has two main options: she can avoid multiplication of a number with a decimal point by converting the amount (0.375 grams) to milligrams (see Chapter 3, Quantity conversions for nurses) and then convert the answer back to grams; or she can multiply 0.375 by 7 and go straight to the answer required.

$$
\begin{array}{r} 0.375 \\ \times\ 7 \\ \hline 2625 \end{array}
\qquad
\begin{array}{|c|}\hline 3 \\ \hline 0 \\ \hline \end{array}
\qquad
\begin{array}{r} 0.375 \\ \times\ 7 \\ \hline 2\ .\ 6\ \ 2\ \ 5 \end{array}
\qquad
\begin{array}{r} 0.375 \\ \times\ 7 \\ \hline 2.625 \end{array}
$$

The placement of the decimal point is often a stumbling block when a multiplication involves decimal points. The easiest way to determine the position of the decimal point in the answer is to count the number of decimal places in the two numbers being multiplied. In the example above, you can see that the top number has three decimal places and the bottom number has zero decimal places. By adding these two values together (and in this case getting three) you can find the correct number of decimal places for the answer. Starting to the right of the last digit, count back the correct number of places (in this case, three) and insert the decimal point. In this example the correct answer is 2.625 grams.

Activity 2.2

As part of a stocktake of drugs at Arcadian Care and Respite Centre, you are to calculate the weekly (7-day) requirement in grams of the prescribed drug dosages for the following patients.

1. Jonathon Sloe needs to have 0.035g per day
2. Jennie Christian needs to have 0.255g per day
3. Steven Grumbles needs to have 5.07g per day

Later on your placement you carry out a similar stocktake at Glad Tidings Rehabilitation Clinic. Again you need to calculate the weekly (7-day) requirement in grams of drugs for the following patients.

4. Freddie Flumpit needs to have 1.45g per day
5. Pauline Poorlie needs to have 0.028g per day
6. Nate Burgen needs to have 3.45g per day
7. Fay Dunnit needs to have 0.020g per day
8. Billy Knotear needs to have 6.5g per day
9. Iama Lookin needs to have 3.75g per day

Division of decimals

Division by whole numbers

The division of a number containing a decimal point can also be done simply because the decimal point in the number being divided will be placed directly above this number. The solution to the task in the following scenario will show you how it is done.

Scenario

Johnson Smilie has been prescribed clemastine fumarate syrup for treatment of his allergic rhinitis. The syrup comes in a bottle containing 75 millilitres. The amount of clemastine fumarate in a bottle of this size is 10.05 milligrams. This is expressed as 10.05mg/75ml on the bottle's label.

You are asked to calculate how many milligrams of clemastine fumarate there are in each millilitre of the syrup. This figure will then be used in later calculations in order to fulfil Johnson's medication requirement.

Given that the bottle contains 75 millilitres, dividing by 75 will reduce the amount to 1 millilitre: any number divided by itself is always 1. The amount of clemastine fumarate in 75 millilitres is 10.05 milligrams. To find the amount of clemastine fumarate in 1ml, you therefore need to divide the drug weight by 75 as well. Making sure that you always divide both the liquid measure and the drug weight by the same number will keep the calculation in balance.

$$\underline{75ml \div 75 \qquad 10.05mg \div 75}$$
$$\triangle$$

This method of calculating the strength per millilitre will be used throughout your nursing career.

In the above scenario you used 75 to reduce the number of millilitres to 1. In the activity that follows you will practise using different liquid volumes. Divide the liquid measure by the total volume to reduce the amount to 1ml, and divide the drug weight by the same number.

> *Hint* ... Always remember to divide both the liquid measure and the drug amount by the same number to keep the calculation balanced.

There will be times when you are dividing numbers and find that you are not able to divide exactly into every digit of the number, or that a digit is too small to be divided. When this occurs, carry that digit or any remainder over to the next available digit in the number being divided. Should you not be able to divide into a digit, remember to place a zero in the answer to indicate this. This method is shown in the first of the diagrams below. The second shows how you would go on to complete the division. The digits and remainders being carried through are shown using smaller digits, written before the next digit in the number being divided. Always continue until the remainder is zero to obtain the correct answer.

$$\begin{array}{r} \boxed{0\ 0.\quad 1} \\ 75\ \overline{\left|1^{1}0.^{10}050\right.} \end{array} \qquad \begin{array}{r} \boxed{0.\quad 1\quad 3\quad 4} \\ 75\ \overline{\left|1^{1}0.^{10}0\ ^{25}5\ ^{30}0\ ^{0}0\right.} \end{array}$$

So 10.05 divided by 75 is equal to 0.134, which tells you each 1 millilitre of syrup contains 0.134 milligrams of weight of the drug. You will use this type of division throughout your career, for example when calculating drug doses or intravenous (IV) flow rates.

Activity 2.3

Calculate the amount of drug weight in 1 millilitre of the following syrup mixtures.

1. 13.2mcg/6ml
2. 57.4mg/7ml
3. 16.5mcg/5ml
4. 2.4g/8ml
5. 2.04mg/4ml
6. 17.6mg/5ml
7. 1.72mcg/4ml
8. 3.25g/5ml
9. 0.072mg/12ml

Division by other decimal values

Should you have to divide a number containing a decimal point by another number that also contains a decimal point, then you need to carry out a preliminary step. Prior to carrying out the division, the number you are dividing by must be made into a whole number. The method of doing this is covered extensively in Chapter 3 (Quantity conversions for nurses) and requires multiplication by 10, 100 or 1000. The number being divided does not need to have its decimal point removed, as seen in the above scenario. However, you must remember to keep things in balance and so you must always multiply both numbers in the calculation by the same value.

Scenario

Mathias Florentino has osteoporosis and will be treated with calcitonin. Mathias's general practitioner (GP) has prescribed 0.09 millilitres of calcitonin per day via a nasal spray. The bottle containing the spray contains 3.6 millilitres. While on placement at the surgery you are asked to work out how many doses of calcitonin Mathias will receive from each bottle of nasal spray.

In order to calculate the number of doses, you need to divide the bottle's contents (3.6ml) by the single dose amount (0.09ml). The number you need to divide by has a decimal point and needs to be made into a whole number prior to the division being carried out. Multiplication by 100 will see the dose 0.09 transformed to become 9. (If you need more detail on this method, see Chapter 3.) To maintain the balance in your calculation you need to do the same to the other value and multiply 3.6 by 100, giving a value of 360.

Hint ... What you do to one side of a calculation you must do to the other.

Now you can divide 360 by 9, obtaining the answer 40. In this case, multiplication by 100 removed the decimal points from both numbers before the division was calculated. However, there is no need to eliminate a decimal point from the number being divided, as shown in the earlier worked example.

Activity 2.4

Work out how many doses of medication can be obtained from the following amounts when divided by the decimal numbers.

1. $27.9 \div 9.0$ 　　　2. $7.5 \div 0.05$ 　　　3. $0.0175 \div 0.05$

4. $15 \div 2.5$ 　　　5. $0.875 \div 0.25$ 　　　6. $0.090 \div 1.6$

Converting fractions to decimals

In Chapter 5 (Drug calculations) you will calculate the doses of medications to be given to patients. One of the potential methods of delivery of this dose is by injection. Since syringes are not marked in fractions you will need to convert any drug amount given as a fraction into a decimal number.

Case study

Showme DeDoor has temporal arteritis, a painful condition. Her doctor has prescribed betamethasone to be administered by the intramuscular route. Her nurse, Yeawhat, has carried out a drug calculation to find the amount of betamethasone injectable suspension to be drawn for the intramuscular injection (IMI). Yeawhat finds it is $\frac{27}{5}$ millilitres which is $5\frac{2}{5}$ millilitres.

Showme's treatment requires her medication to be injected and so Yeawhat needs the answer in decimal format. Hypodermic syringes are always marked in decimal format and never in fractions, so the amount of liquid in every injection given will need to be converted to decimal format for all non-whole-number answers. This can be done prior to cancelling ($\frac{27}{5}$ in this scenario) or using the final result ($5\frac{2}{5}$ here). In either case, you obtain the whole number 5; the fraction $\frac{2}{5}$ indicates a remainder of 2 still to be divided by 5.

Hint ... To convert any fraction to a decimal you divide the top number by the bottom number.

In this example the top number in the fraction ($\frac{2}{5}$ or $\frac{27}{5}$) does not have a decimal point, so you need to place one directly behind the last digit. You can now divide the top number by the bottom number to find the decimal value.

$$\boxed{0.4}$$
$$5\,\overline{)2.\,^20\,^00}$$

$$\boxed{5.4}$$
$$5\,\overline{)2\,^27.\,^20\,^00}$$

When the fraction $\frac{2}{5}$ is converted to a decimal the result is 0.4, which is then added to the whole number 5 to give the final answer, 5.4 millilitres.

If you choose to convert to a decimal from the fraction $\frac{27}{5}$ you should obtain the answer 5.4ml in one step. Notice that both answers are the same, and accurate.

So for Showme's IMI, Yeawhat will need to draw up 5.4 millilitres of betamethasone.

Activity 2.5

These 12 fractions are drug doses that you have calculated for patients. Now you need to convert the results to decimal answers, as all the medications are to be injected.

1. $\frac{17}{2}$ 2. $\frac{13}{4}$ 3. $\frac{7}{2}$ 4. $\frac{18}{8}$

5. $\frac{26}{5}$ 6. $\frac{175}{100}$ 7. $\frac{375}{25}$ 8. $\frac{4}{5}$

9. $\frac{12}{5}$ 10. $\frac{102}{15}$ 11. $\frac{77}{35}$ 12. $\frac{87}{30}$

Converting decimals to fractions

There will be times when an order is given to a nurse as a decimal, but it would be quicker to complete the task using a fraction, as in the following scenario.

Scenario

Kiefer Da Door has had a fall from his bicycle and grazed his lower arm and elbow. His injury is not thought to be serious but may require sutures. Prior to Kiefer's assessment by the Charge Nurse, you have been asked to prepare an iodine solution to clean the wound to remove any loose skin. The solution strength required is 0.2 parts iodine mixed with sterile water.

Kiefer's injury is to be cleaned using a solution you must prepare. The solution strength is to be 0.2 parts iodine mixed with sterile water. Before you can calculate the amounts required you will need to convert 0.2 to a fraction. This fraction will then show what proportion of the total will be iodine in the mixed solution.

The conversion process is among the easiest you will encounter. To write the decimal as a fraction, use the decimal as the numerator (or top digit/s); the denominator (or bottom digit/s) will be a multiple of 10 (10, 100, 1000 ...) and can be found by counting the number of decimal places.

In the scenario, Kiefer's mixture was 0.2 and so the numerator will be 2. Notice that the decimal point has now been dropped. Since the decimal has just one place, there will be one zero in the denominator.

As a fraction 0.2 is $\frac{2}{10}$, which can be cancelled down to $\frac{1}{5}$.

This fraction will allow you to mix the solution to clean Kiefer's wounds. Since the order was for 0.2 iodine solution and you have now calculated this to be $\frac{1}{5}$, you know that any solution used is to be $\frac{1}{5}$ iodine plus $\frac{4}{5}$ sterile water.

> *Hint* ... To convert from a fraction to a decimal, use the decimal digits as the numerator, and the number 1 followed by as many zeros as decimal places for the denominator.

Activity 2.6

Convert the following decimals to fractions in their simplest or lowest form.

1. 0.05	2. 0.075	3. 0.35	4. 0.025
5. 0.84	6. 0.375	7. 0.02	8. 0.045
9. 0.605	10. 0.875	11. 0.700	12. 0.65

Rounding decimals and fractions

When you are calculating the flow rate of an IV infusion for your patient (as in Chapter 6, Calculating intravenous rates), the answer needs to be a whole number because a droplet cannot be successfully divided. You therefore need to be able to round to the nearest whole number.

> ## Scenario
>
> ....
>
> Following a surgical procedure your patient, Katz Whiskars, is to have an IV infusion. You have accurately calculated the flow rate using the formula from Chapter 6 and found it to be $41\frac{3}{5}$ or, as a decimal, 41.6 drops per minute. You must now determine the correct number of drops per minute.

Without the correct flow rate, Katz could receive her IV infusion too quickly, or may not receive her total medication in the prescribed time period. Either case could have serious consequences.

To decide whether to round up or down, simply judge if the fraction or decimal has reached or passed half way. If your answer is a decimal, look at the first number after the decimal point. If this number is 5 or greater, then the number before the decimal point should be increased to the next whole number. The decimal point and every number beyond it are then deleted.

If your answer is a whole number plus a fraction, look at the fraction. If the numerator (top number) of the fraction is half or more of the denominator (bottom number), then the whole number should be increased to the next number. The fraction is then deleted from your answer.

For answers where the decimal or fractions do not reach half way or greater, then the decimal or fraction is simply deleted from the answer and the whole number is not changed.

> *Hint* ... If the decimal is 0.5 or larger, or the fraction $\frac{1}{2}$ or larger, then the whole number value increases to the next whole number value and the decimal or fraction is deleted. If the decimal or fraction is less than half, the whole number value remains unchanged and the decimal or fraction is deleted.

In the scenario above, Katz's IV rate was calculated at $41\frac{3}{5}$ or 41.6 drops per minute. The fraction $\frac{3}{5}$ is greater than $\frac{1}{2}$ and the decimal 0.6 is greater than 0.5. So when you set the flow rate for Katz's IV you will set it at 42 drops/minute.

In preparation for later chapters in this book, attempt the following activity on rounding of fractions and decimals.

Activity 2.7

Round each of the following values to the nearest whole number.

1. 3.7	2. $12\frac{5}{8}$	3. 7.7	4. $15\frac{2}{9}$
5. 5.2	6. $25\frac{8}{17}$	7. 32.09	8. $44\frac{8}{9}$
9. 17.6	10. 1.16	11. $24\frac{3}{7}$	12. 8.93
13. $1\frac{17}{32}$	14. 5.3	15. 45.53	

Converting time fractions and decimals to minutes

There will be times when the number of hours over which a medication or treatment is to be given is not in whole hours. For example, on your placement you may encounter a patient having chemotherapy whose treatment does not take an exact number of whole hours.

Scenario

Rusty Bouquets is undergoing chemotherapy at the respite centre where you are currently on placement. Rusty is to receive his medication using a volumetric pump and it will be delivered over a period of $3\frac{1}{3}$ hours. Rusty wants to know how many hours and minutes the volumetric pump will take for the infusion so he can arrange transport home.

Details of how to calculate the length of time taken are covered in Chapter 6 (Calculating intravenous rates); here we shall concentrate on the conversion of the time fraction.

To convert a time fraction to a number of minutes, multiply the fraction by 60. Since there are 60 minutes in one hour, this will give the exact number of minutes equal to the fraction of an hour. For Rusty this means $\frac{1}{3} \times 60$ which you can cancel down using skills learnt earlier in this chapter.

$$\frac{1}{\cancel{3}} \times \frac{\cancel{60}}{1} = \frac{1}{1} \times \frac{20}{1} = \frac{20}{1} = 20 \text{ minutes}$$

You can now accurately say that the volumetric pump will take 3 hours and 20 minutes to infuse Rusty's chemotherapy medication and he can book his transportation home.

If the result is in decimal format, then multiply the decimal by 60, again because there are 60 minutes in one hour. Multiplying a decimal was covered earlier in this chapter should you wish to review it.

Scenario

Chris Wakim is receiving light treatment for a skin condition. The consultant has prescribed 2.6 hours under the treatment light for Chris. You are the primary carer for this treatment and must calculate the number of hours and minutes of its duration.

To convert a time decimal to minutes, multiply the decimal by 60. Since there are 60 minutes in one hour this will give the exact number of minutes equal to the decimal.

$0.6 \times 60 = 36.0$ minutes

So the number of hours and minutes will be 2 hours 36 minutes. To convert the total time to minutes you could multiply the whole number by 60.

$2.6 \times 60 = 156.0$ minutes

Activity 2.8

Convert the following fractions of hours to a number of minutes.

1. $\dfrac{4}{5}$ 2. $\dfrac{2}{3}$ 3. $\dfrac{6}{5}$ 4. $\dfrac{9}{4}$

5. $\dfrac{7}{2}$ 6. $\dfrac{3}{10}$ 7. $\dfrac{5}{15}$ 8. $\dfrac{12}{60}$

Convert the following hours, shown as decimals, to a total number of minutes.

1. 2.35   2. 3.2   3. 0.8   4. 0.6

5. 0.15   6. 0.05   7. 16.05   8. 0.025

9. 4.7   10. 3.05   11. 6.05   12. 1.3

Addition and subtraction

Most student nurses take it for granted that they can carry out addition and subtraction. Your patients and colleagues will rely on your ability to carry out these tasks accurately. In Chapter 4 (Fluid balance and maintenance) you will use your addition and subtraction skills to calculate your patient's **fluid balance**. The fluid balance is the amount of fluid the patient is retaining to ensure their hydration levels are sufficient to maintain life.

Addition

Scenario

You are currently calculating the fluid balance for Sergeant Major Boris who has been recorded as having consumed the following liquids: tea 800ml, coffee 550ml, water 600ml and juice 175ml over a 24-hour period. You have to calculate Sergeant Major Boris's total fluid intake for the day as part of your daily duties, an NMC professional standard requirement (29(ii)).

In order to find the total amount of fluid, you need to add all the amounts of different fluids consumed. The best-practice method is to list the numbers one above the other. Keeping the digits in alignment allows you to total each column of numbers in turn. Should a column total become double digits, place the first digit at the base of the next column to the left. The second digit goes into the total as part of the answer sought.

$$\begin{array}{r} 175 \\ 600 \\ 550 \\ 800 \\ 1 \\ \hline 2125\text{ml} \end{array}$$

You can now confidently report on his Fluid Balance Chart that the Sergeant Major has consumed 2125ml of fluid on this day.

Subtraction

Scenario

You are currently calculating the fluid balance for Corporal Norty. He has been recorded as having consumed 2125ml of liquids on the day being charted. His total **fluid output** was recorded as 1960ml. To complete the chart you must now subtract the output from the input to obtain the fluid balance.

As for addition, align the digits of the numbers above each other. When a value being subtracted is too large to be subtracted from the digit above it, you will need to 'borrow' from the digit to the left in the top number. This will lower the value you borrow from by 1, as can be seen in the diagram, and increase the digit you are subtracting from by 10. These changes are shown using small digits.

$$\begin{array}{cccc} {}^1\!\!\not{2} & {}^{10}\!\!\not{+} & {}^1\!\!\not{2} & 5 \\ 1 & 9 & 6 & 0 \\ \hline 0 & 1 & 6 & 5\text{ml} \end{array}$$

The result gives Corporal Norty a fluid balance of 165ml for the day on which the figures were recorded.

> *Hint* ... You should always subtract the lesser value number from the greater value number. Should the amount expended (output) be more than the amount consumed (intake), this would indicate a negative fluid balance.

A negative balance should be preceded by the word 'Minus' or clearly marked with the – symbol.

Activity 2.9

The following patients are all under observation. For each patient, find the total fluid intake, the total fluid output, and hence the fluid balance.

1. Jackson Dunnit consumed the following:
   235ml + 125ml + 175ml + 480ml
   The following amounts were recorded as outputs:
   275ml + 157ml + 345ml + 165ml

2. Ed Wazzear consumed the following:
   315ml + 380ml + 275ml + 220ml
   The following amounts were recorded as outputs:
   295ml + 165ml + 153ml + 225ml

3. Ali Barba consumed the following:
   485ml + 575ml + 175ml + 376ml
   The following amounts were recorded as outputs:
   450ml + 525ml + 315ml + 375ml

Chapter summary

Patients rely on nurses to accurately calculate their medications as prescribed. Later in this book we will guide you through that skill. In order to do this as part of your duties you must first be able to master the mathematical skills shown in this chapter. The methods and skills you practise and become proficient at here will enable you to become a mathematically proficient nurse.

This chapter is one of the major building blocks on which your nursing career is built and you should feel comfortable doing all the activities provided. Students are often anxious about the mathematics in use throughout nursing because complete accuracy is essential. This anxiety is misplaced, since with practice and by using this book you will gain confidence and realise the simplicity of the calculations required in nursing. Throughout this book, and indeed throughout your career, you can always refer back to this chapter if you need to refresh your memory/skills.

Useful websites

For free online guides and resources on basic mathematics revision, refer to the following websites.

BBC Bitesize and Skillswise

The BBC Bitesize and Skillswise websites offer many tutorials which could be used to gain more practice at a basic mathematics level.

1. Times tables grid

    www.bbc.co.uk/education/topics/znmtsbk

2. Multiplication methods

    www.bbc.co.uk/education/topics/znmtsbk

3. Long multiplication and division

    www.bbc.co.uk/schools/gcsebitesize/maths/number/multiplicationdivisionrev1. shtml

4. Division using repeated subtraction

    www.bbc.co.uk/education/topics/znmtsbk

5. Rounding

    www.bbc.co.uk/schools/gcsebitesize/maths/number/roundestimaterev2.shtml

6. Addition

   www.bbc.co.uk/education/topics/znmtsbk

7. Subtraction

   www.bbc.co.uk/education/topics/znmtsbk

OpenLearn

8. Numbers, units and arithmetic

   http://labspace.open.ac.uk/course/view.php?id=3434

9. Rounding and estimation

   http://labspace.open.ac.uk/course/view.php?id=3586

Visit the online resources on your computer at **https://study.sagepub.com/starkings krause4e** or on your smart phone or tablet and gain access to:

- over 400 extra questions to check your learning and gain extra practice;
- links to useful websites that build on the skills introduced in this chapter;
- an interactive glossary of key terms.

Answers to the activities

Activity 2.1 (pages 19–20)

1. $\dfrac{675}{900} = \dfrac{3}{4}$　　2. $\dfrac{400}{850} = \dfrac{8}{17}$　　3. $\dfrac{5}{75} = \dfrac{1}{15}$　　4. $\dfrac{6}{104} = \dfrac{3}{52}$

5. $\dfrac{17}{51} = \dfrac{1}{3}$　　6. $\dfrac{16}{96} = \dfrac{1}{6}$　　7. $\dfrac{3}{75} = \dfrac{1}{25}$　　8. $\dfrac{75}{300} = \dfrac{1}{4}$

9. $\dfrac{13}{104} = \dfrac{1}{8}$　　10. $\dfrac{96}{480} = \dfrac{1}{5}$　　11. $\dfrac{228}{528} = \dfrac{19}{44}$　　12. $\dfrac{35}{85} = \dfrac{7}{17}$

You can revise your times tables using one of the useful websites listed, or any other appropriate source. The ability to cancel down is a skill every nurse can use to make the calculation of drug doses easier to carry out accurately.

Activity 2.2 (page 21)

Weekly requirement = Daily requirement × 7

Therefore the patients' requirements for 7 days will be as follows.

1. Jonathon Sloe needs to have 0.035g per day so for 7 days needs 0.245g

2. Jennie Christian needs to have 0.255g per day so for 7 days needs 1.785g

3. Steven Grumbles needs to have 5.07g per day so for 7 days needs 35.49g

4. Freddie Flumpit needs to have 1.45g per day so for 7 days needs 10.15g

5. Pauline Poorlie needs to have 0.028g per day so for 7 days needs 0.196g

6. Nate Burgen needs to have 3.45g per day so for 7 days needs 24.15g

7. Fay Dunnit needs to have 0.020g per day so for 7 days needs 0.14g

8. Billy Knotear needs to have 6.5g per day so for 7 days needs 45.5g

9. Iama Lookin needs to have 3.75g per day so for 7 days needs 26.25g

Accuracy is what every nurse strives to achieve at all times. The ability to multiply numbers containing a decimal point accurately is essential.

Activity 2.3 (page 23)

The amount of drug weight in 1 millilitre of the syrup mixtures is as follows.

1. 2.2mcg/ml	2. 8.2mg/ml	3. 3.3mcg/ml
4. 0.3g/ml	5. 0.51mg/ml	6. 3.52mg/ml
7. 0.43mcg/ml	8. 0.65g/ml	9. 0.006mg/ml

This activity enables you to practise your division and cancelling down methods, skills which every nurse could use many times in their daily duties.

Activity 2.4 (page 24)

The numbers of doses of medication obtained from the amounts are as follows.

1. $27.9 \div 9.0 = 3.1$
2. $7.5 \div 0.05 = 150$
3. $0.0175 \div 0.05 = 0.35$
4. $15 \div 2.5 = 6$
5. $0.875 \div 0.25 = 3.5$
6. $0.090 \div 1.6 = 0.05625$

Activity 2.5 (page 25)

To convert any fraction to a decimal, you divide the number on the top by the number on the bottom.

1. $\dfrac{17}{2} = 8.5$
2. $\dfrac{13}{4} = 3.25$
3. $\dfrac{7}{2} = 3.5$
4. $\dfrac{18}{8} = 2.25$

5. $\dfrac{26}{5} = 5.2$
6. $\dfrac{175}{100} = 1.75$
7. $\dfrac{375}{25} = 15$
8. $\dfrac{4}{5} = 0.8$

9. $\dfrac{12}{15} = 0.8$
10. $\dfrac{102}{15} = 6.8$
11. $\dfrac{77}{35} = 2.2$
12. $\dfrac{87}{30} = 2.9$

Activity 2.6 (page 26)

To convert from a fraction to a decimal, use the decimal digits as the numerator and the number 1 followed by as many zeros as decimal places for the denominator. Then use your skills in cancelling down to obtain the simplest or lowest form.

1. $0.05 = \dfrac{5}{100} = \dfrac{1}{20}$

2. $0.075 = \dfrac{75}{1000} = \dfrac{3}{40}$

3. $0.35 = \dfrac{35}{100} = \dfrac{7}{20}$

4. $0.025 = \dfrac{25}{1000} = \dfrac{1}{40}$

5. $0.84 = \dfrac{84}{100} = \dfrac{21}{25}$

6. $0.375 = \dfrac{375}{1000} = \dfrac{3}{8}$

7. $0.02 = \dfrac{2}{100} = \dfrac{1}{50}$

8. $0.045 = \dfrac{45}{1000} = \dfrac{9}{200}$

9. $0.605 = \dfrac{605}{1000} = \dfrac{121}{200}$

10. $0.875 = \dfrac{875}{1000} = \dfrac{7}{8}$

11. $0.700 = \dfrac{700}{1000} = \dfrac{7}{10}$

12. $0.65 = \dfrac{65}{100} = \dfrac{13}{20}$

Activity 2.7 (page 28)

If the decimal is equal to or greater than 0.5 or the fraction equal to or greater than $\dfrac{1}{2}$, then the whole number is increased to the next whole number.

1. $3.7 \rightarrow 4$

2. $12\dfrac{5}{8} \rightarrow 13$

3. $7.7 \rightarrow 8$

4. $15\dfrac{2}{9} \rightarrow 15$

5. $5.2 \rightarrow 5$

6. $25\dfrac{8}{17} \rightarrow 25$

7. $32.09 \rightarrow 32$

8. $44\dfrac{8}{9} \rightarrow 45$

9. $17.6 \rightarrow 18$

10. $1.16 \rightarrow 1$

11. $24\dfrac{3}{7} \rightarrow 24$

12. $8.93 \rightarrow 9$

13. $1\dfrac{17}{32} \rightarrow 2$

14. $5.3 \rightarrow 5$

15. $45.53 \rightarrow 46$

Activity 2.8 (page 29)

To convert a time fraction to a number of minutes, multiply the fraction by 60.

1. $\dfrac{4}{5} = 48$

2. $\dfrac{2}{3} = 40$

3. $\dfrac{6}{5} = 72$

4. $\dfrac{9}{4} = 135$

5. $\dfrac{7}{2} = 210$

6. $\dfrac{3}{10} = 18$

7. $\dfrac{5}{15} = 20$

8. $\dfrac{12}{60} = 12$

To convert the total time to minutes, multiply the number by 60.

1. $2.35 = 141$

2. $3.2 = 192$

3. $0.8 = 48$

4. $0.6 = 36$

5. $0.15 = 9$

6. $0.05 = 3$

7. $16.05 = 963$

8. $0.025 = 1.5$

9. $4.7 = 282$

10. $3.05 = 183$

11. $6.05 = 363$

12. $1.3 = 78$

Activity 2.9 (page 31)

1. Jackson Dunnit consumed the following:

    235ml + 125ml + 175ml + 480ml

    The following amounts were recorded as outputs:

    275ml + 157ml + 345ml + 165ml

    1015 − 942 = A positive balance of 73ml

2. Ed Wazzear consumed the following:

    315ml + 380ml + 275ml + 220ml

    The following amounts were recorded as outputs:

    295ml + 165ml + 153ml + 225ml

    1190 − 838 = A positive balance of 352ml

3. Ali Barba consumed the following:

    485ml + 575ml + 175ml + 376ml

    The following amounts were recorded as outputs:

    450ml + 525ml + 315ml + 375ml

    1611 − 1665 = A negative balance of 54ml

Chapter 3

Quantity conversions for nurses

Chapter aims

By the end of this chapter you should be able to:

- convert a given weight, be it of a drug or a person, into a greater or lesser metric unit of weight;
- convert a liquid measure from litres to millilitres and from millilitres to litres;
- convert a given measurement of length into a lesser or greater metric unit of length;
- multiply any amount by 10, 100, 1000.

Introduction

In this chapter you will find examples of the kind of calculations you will need to make in converting units of metric measurement. Throughout your career as a nurse you will need to convert these measures in order to be able to make calculations before administering medications. The patient's prescription could be listed in milligrams, while the drug available at your placement is listed in grams. Before you can accurately calculate the patient's requirement, you will need to convert either the amount needed or the available stock so that they use the same unit of measure.

Hint ... The ability to convert metric measures is essential in healthcare; without it, the patient may receive an incorrect dose of medication. Inaccuracy could lead to an accidental overdose of the drug. This could be as much as 1000 times too much. The all-too-frequent mistakes reported as tragedies in the news reinforce the need for accuracy in all your calculations.

Your skill in accurately converting metric measurements will be examined in many formats; for example, in a formative test done without the use of a calculator or as part of a larger scenario question. Such a question may involve a patient prescribed a number of different drugs, some of which require their measures of strength to be converted prior to calculation of their dosage.

You may need to convert a patient's weight or height in order to compare it with a standardised body mass index chart to check for indications of obesity. As in all chapters, it is suggested that you do the activities without the aid of a calculator in order to become more proficient.

Practising liquid, weight and length conversions will help you, as the future nurse, develop the skills to become more confident with the conversions needed. This chapter will cover the various best-practice methods for the types of conversions that nurses will encounter and perform during their careers.

In Figure 3.1, units of liquid measurement are shown on the left, and units of weight measurement on the right (there is no relationship between liquid measures and weight, except that 1ml of water weighs 1g).

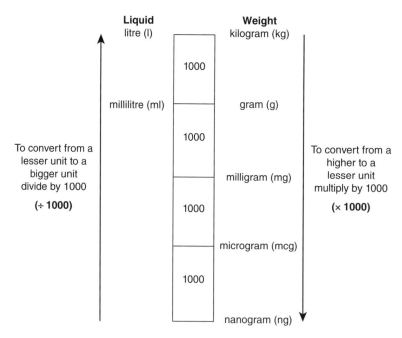

Figure 3.1 Weights and liquids ladder of conversion

Notice that the abbreviation for litre is the small letter l; be careful not to confuse this with the numeral 1.

If you look at the top of the ladder you will see that the largest unit of weight is a kilogram (kg) and the largest commonly used unit for liquids is a litre (l).

The kilogram can be divided up into 1000 units, each of which is known as a gram (g). The gram can then be divided into 1000 units, each being called a milligram (mg).

The milligram can then be divided into 1000 units, each of which is a microgram (mcg). Those studying children's nursing will also need to know that the microgram is also divisible into 1000 units, each of which is known as a nanogram (ng). The nanogram is generally seen only in conjunction with children's medical requirements because of the very small size of the metric unit of weight involved. Chapter 7 (Calculations and children) covers smaller dosages in more detail. Great care should be taken not to confuse similar abbreviations when using abbreviations of measurements. See page 3 for more details.

Each litre can be divided into 1000 parts, each of which is called a millilitre (ml). This is as low as a litre is currently divided in most nursing and healthcare situations.

The distance between each rung on the ladder in Figure 3.1 is 1000 units. So we can say there is a 'factor of 1000' between the metric units most commonly used for liquid and weight measures by nurses. The easiest way to handle conversions between these units is to use this fact and simply multiply or divide by 1000, as shown in Figure 3.1 and in the activities that follow.

Metric units of length are converted differently, and are discussed later in the chapter.

Calculating from one unit to another

Look again at Figure 3.1. On each side of the ladder are instructions about converting between units using either multiplication or division. For example, if you want to convert millilitres to litres, the arrow shows that you have to divide by 1000.

An easy way to do this is to move the decimal point. The number of times the decimal point moves is dictated by the number of zeros in the factor. In the number 1000 there are three zeros, so the point must move three places.

The arrows on either side of the ladder in Figure 3.1 are there to help you remember in which direction to move the decimal point. To convert liquid and weight measures you will always use a factor of 1000, so all you need to decide is whether to move the decimal point to the left or right. Suppose you are required to convert down, from a larger unit to a smaller unit (such as from kilograms to grams); this conversion moves *down* the ladder, and the down arrow is on the *right*. This reminds you to move the decimal point three places to the right.

Multiplying by 1000

00   0   0.0

You can convert units using this method whether you are changing litres to millilitres or milligrams to micrograms. If the unit you wish to convert from appears above the unit you wish to convert to in the ladder of conversion, then you need to multiply by 1000. You will move the decimal point three places to the *right*; hence the arrow to remind you is on the *right* of the ladder.

Dividing by 1000

There may be times during your training and later in your career where you are called upon to convert a measure upwards. It could be that a patient's fluid balance is being recorded on their chart. Their drink container is marked in millilitres but the information is to be recorded in litres on the chart. In this scenario you would need to go *up* the ladder and the up arrow is on the *left*. The decimal point must go *left* as you need to divide the amount you have in millilitres to obtain the measurement in litres.

For both multiplication and division by 1000, the decimal point will move three places from its original position.

Should a number have no decimal point, then you would start from behind the last digit. In the number 75 there is currently no decimal point showing. However, you can write in the decimal point directly after the last digit, and add some zeros in readiness for conversion, giving, for example, 75.00. If a number already has a decimal point, you should always start your conversion from there; if there are not enough digits to complete the process, you can always add zeros to the front or back of a number before starting to move the decimal point. This will ensure you have no empty spaces when the conversion is completed.

So far we have been multiplying and dividing by 1000. Later in the chapter you will need to multiply or divide by 10 and 100. The number 10 has one zero and so requires a move of just one place, and 100 has two zeros and so the decimal point will move two places: to the left for division or to the right for multiplication.

Scenario

Oar Sum suffers from gastroesophageal reflux disease and has been ordered 20mg of omeprazole to be given orally. As Oar's nurse you have checked the medication available on the ward (stock on hand) and found that the dispensed dose is 0.04g per tablet. Before you can calculate how many tablets Oar will need to take (covered in Chapter 5, Drug calculations), you must convert the units of either the stock on hand (currently in grams) or the ordered amount (currently in milligrams) so that they are both in the same units.

You need to change the units in 0.04g (the stock tablets) to milligrams (mg), to match the units used for the prescribed amount. Converting to the smaller unit will eliminate the decimal point. Putting both the stock required (need) and the stock on hand (have) in the same units means that when you cancel down, as seen in Chapter 2, the 'need' and 'have' unit measures of the drug calculation will cancel each other, leaving just the stock unit measure for your dosage.

$$\frac{\text{Need } \cancel{mg}}{\text{Have } \cancel{mg}} \times \frac{\text{Stock (Unit Measure)}}{1}$$

Let's use Figure 3.1 to do the conversion. Since milligrams (mg) lie below grams (g) on the ladder, then the conversion is to be done using the down arrow, which is on the right, meaning that we have to move the decimal point to the right. So we start with 0.04 and move the decimal point three places to the right:

0 0 4 0·0

Notice that there were insufficient zeros at the end of the number to complete the conversion, and so two extra zeros have been added.

You now know that the omeprazole tablets on hand are of strength 40.0mg and can accurately calculate the number of tablets required. The last zero and the decimal point can be deleted as they serve no purpose; the tablets are 40mg strength.

Scenario

Wily Olfox has ulcerative colitis and has been ordered 0.75mg of mesalamine to be given orally. Stock on hand is 250mcg capsules. You need to find the strength of mesalamine capsules that Willy should be given in mcg.

Since micrograms (mcg) lie below milligrams (mg) on the ladder (Figure 3.1), the conversion will be done using the down arrow, which is on the right, so you need to move the decimal point to the right.

0 7 5 0.0

Again, as there were insufficient places into which to move the point, an extra two zeros were added to 0.75 before the conversion was completed. It is now clear that the amount of mesalamine ordered for Mr Olfox is 750.0mcg. Again, the final zero and the decimal point can now be deleted, so the answer is 750mcg.

Now try the following activity to see if you understand how to use the method employed in the scenarios to calculate a conversion. You need to make a conversion so that both stock strength (what you *have*) and stock required (what you *need*) are in the same units. You should try the activities without the aid of a calculator.

Activity 3.1

Commonly used as an anticoagulant, warfarin helps to prevent clots in veins, arteries, the lungs or heart. At the Yew Tree Retirement Day Care and Respite Play Arena it is kept in the medicine cabinet in various stock strength tablets. Patients under your care are being treated with this drug and will be taking their medication daily. At the start of your shift you need to calculate the number of milligrams required for the following patients.

1. Jennie Snoozars needs to have 0.070g
2. Mitch Crump needs to have 0.015g
3. Hermany Crusty needs to have 0.35g

There are many treatments for hypertension, one of which is the drug prazosin. At the Ol Geezer's Rehabilitation Clinic the following clients are being treated with this drug and will be taking their dosage once a day. The clinical supervisor has tasked you with calculating the number of milligrams required for the following clients.

4. Walla B needs to have 475mcg
5. Ken Garo needs to have 0.04g
6. Nickola Surgeon needs to have 1750mcg
7. Adi Nahwaz needs to have 1.02g
8. Andy Ritt needs to have 750mcg
9. Notta Clue needs to have 0.0205g

Answers to all activities can be found at the end of the chapter.

Converting dosages involving mixtures

In the previous section you learnt how to convert units of weight for tablets or capsules. In this section we will look at the conversion of drug weights found in medications comprising mixtures and syrups.

Scenario

Wattle, a patient under your care on Banksia Cancer Ward, has been prescribed panitumumab 75mg to slow the growth of her cancer cells. The dispensed dose available on the ward is in a liquid mixture containing 0.1g of drug per 5ml, expressed as 0.1g/5ml. As Wattle's nurse, you need to work out how many milligrams there are in each 5ml in order to allow correct calculation of the dosage to be given to Wattle.

To find out how many milligrams of drug there are in 5ml of a mixture with a strength of 0.1g/5ml you will need to refer back to Figure 3.1. You will need to add extra zeros to the number to provide places for the decimal point to move to. According to the ladder, converting grams to milligrams is *down*, so move the decimal point to the *right*.

The strength in milligram per 5ml mixture is:

0 1   0 0 . 0

You have to move the decimal point three places to the right as indicated by the ladder. The panitumumab strength is 100mg per 5ml, expressed as 100mg/5ml.

The ladder shown in Figure 3.1 can be used to convert metric units of measure for any drug, whatever form it comes in.

> *Hint* ... A general best-practice rule is to always convert to the smaller unit when dealing with two different weight measures.

If you are dealing with both grams and milligrams, then convert both to milligrams as in the scenario above.

Remember that in a liquid mixture or syrup, only the weight component requires conversion as the liquid volume will always remain the same figure as given.

Activity 3.2

1. Justin is under your care and has been ordered 0.095g of penicillin orally. What is the required amount of penicillin in milligrams for Justin's dose?

(Continued)

(Continued)

2. Matthew has been prescribed flucloxacillin. The stock suspension is 1.25g/5ml. What is the stock strength of the medication in mg/ml?
3. Askme has a mild infection and has been ordered benzyl penicillin from an available mixture of 0.24g/3ml. What is this strength in mg/ml?
4. Flatulance has been ordered paracetamol, and the stock syrup on hand is 0.35g/7ml. What is this strength in mg/ml?

Activity 3.3

Sertraline is an antidepressant, one of a group of drugs called selective serotonin reuptake inhibitors (SSRIs). Your current placement sees you working in a mental health outpatient clinic and as part of their treatment several service users have been prescribed sertraline to ease their symptoms.

Calculate the following amounts in milligrams for these service users.

1. Didya Dunnit is prescribed a dose of 0.05g
2. Jose Thisa is prescribed a dose of 0.085g
3. Marie Mevicar is prescribed a dose of 75mcg

Pethidine is an analgesic used to ease pain during childbirth. During a placement at a birthing centre attached to the regional hospital you are assisting in the care of the following women. They have been prescribed a single dose of pethidine by the Non-Medical Prescribing (NMP) Nurse in charge at the centre.

Calculate the amount required in micrograms for the following new mothers.

4. Leif Blowhard is prescribed a dose of 0.17mg
5. Dunnit Argan is prescribed a dose of 0.705mg
6. Ruby Rose is prescribed a dose of 0.675mg

A powerful steroidal anti-inflammatory drug in common use is cortisone. During a placement at Krabbies Retirement and Care Village you will be caring for the following residents, who have mild to severe arthritis and have been prescribed cortisone to ease their pain.

Calculate the amount ordered in milligrams for the following residents.

7. Argus Tuft is prescribed a dose of 675mcg
8. Wasit Youse is prescribed a dose of 0.035g
9. Well Inever is prescribed a dose of 0.2g

Conversion of body weight

At times drug doses may be ordered based on a patient's body weight; this is often the case with children's doses and will be covered in further detail in Chapter 7. Drugs could be ordered in micrograms, milligrams or grams per kilogram per day, which may then be divided up into a number of single doses. So if your patient's personal chart has their weight recorded in grams, you will need to convert this amount to kilograms prior to commencing any calculations for their medication.

Scenario

Edmund Lilycrapper has been prescribed erythromycin. The dosage prescribed is 4mg/kg/day, four doses daily. Edmund was weighed on Popkorn Ward today and recorded at 16500g. Before you can determine the correct dosage Edmund requires, you must convert his recorded weight to kilograms. This will then allow the calculations to be done (as shown in Chapter 5, Drug calculations and Chapter 7, Calculations and children).

To find out how much Edmund weighs in kilograms you again refer to the ladder in Figure 3.1. The weight is in grams and is required in kilograms, which necessitates going up the ladder, and therefore dividing by 1000. Therefore you need to move the decimal point three places to the left.

16.5 0 0

So Edmund weighs 16.5kg; as the final zeros have no bearing on the number, they can be deleted. From this information it is now possible to calculate the amount of erythromycin Edmund requires.

Activity 3.4

To help treat infection, particularly after an operation, chloramphenicol is at times given to patients. The following patients on Hibiscus Ward have been ordered chloramphenicol and individual doses will be calculated according to the patient's body weight. Express the following patients' weights in kilograms.

1. Digger Hole weighs 61 035g
2. Shaz Ham weighs 5700g
3. Jerry Mander weighs 3247g

(Continued)

(Continued)

4. Alex Uburk weighs 637g
5. Betty Mustgo weighs 1957g

Express the following patients' weights in grams.

6. Cerius Lee weighs 2.807kg
7. Philip Eans weighs 0.108kg
8. Ya Watt weighs 37.63kg
9. Ash Ford weighs 24.07kg
10. Well Iwood weighs 6.405kg

Conversion of metric units in length

The basic metric unit of length is the metre which, like all other metric units, can be divided into smaller units such as the centimetre and millimetre.

The units of length most often used by nurses are metres and centimetres. A metre can be divided into 100 parts, each of which is a centimetre. A metre can also be divided into 1000 parts, with each part known as a millimetre. The millimetre is also equivalent to one-tenth of a centimetre. As with the metric measures used for liquid and weight, the easiest way to illustrate the relationship between metric length measures is with a ladder, as shown in Figure 3.2.

Scenario

Sigmund has arrived on the Kornie Ward and as part of the admission process his height was measured at 1.15m. You have been asked to convert his height into centimetres. This height, along with his previously taken weight measure, will then be used on the Body Mass Index and Growth charts currently being used by the paediatric department to chart his development.

In the nursing environment you could come across metric length measures in any of the three units shown in Figure 3.2.

Converting metres to centimetres

To find out how tall Sigmund is in centimetres refer to Figure 3.2. Given a height in metres and requiring it in centimetres means you have to move down the ladder, multiplying by 100. As seen in previous conversion activities, multiplying moves the decimal

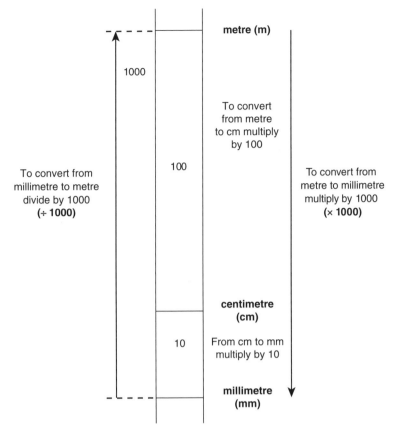

Figure 3.2 Conversion of length in metric units

point to the right. Unlike weight and liquid conversions, where a factor of 1000 was universal, here the factor is 100, so you move the point by only two places.

> *Hint* ... Move the decimal point three places for the factor 1000, which has three zeros, only two places for the factor 100 as it has only two zeros, and only one place for 10 as it has only one zero.

1.15m expressed in centimetres is 115cm.

Converting centimetres to millimetres

If any length given in centimetres is required in millimetres, such as for use on a growth chart, you can again use the ladder for the conversion. The direction is down, as before, but this time only by a factor of 10. The conversion involves moving the decimal point one place to the right, as 10 has only one zero.

1 1 5 0 . 0

In this example, there were insufficient digits in the number to complete the conversion so extra zeros were added to 115. The result is that 115cm is equal to 1150mm.

Converting metres to millimetres

The use of growth charts is extensive in children's nursing and some of these charts will require length measures in millimetres. You can use the ladder (Figure 3.2) to convert Sigmund's height directly from metres to millimetres; the factor is 1000. The conversion therefore involves moving the decimal point three places to the right, as 1000 has three zeros.

1 1 5 0 . 0

This confirms that Sigmund's height in millimetres is 1150mm.

Scenario

Seven Wongs on Norty Ward had her height measured at 1026mm. As an exercise, you have been asked to convert it from millimetres to both centimetres and metres.

Converting from millimetres to metres

To convert Seven's height, given in millimetres, to metres, you need to use the ladder in Figure 3.2, this time going upwards. Converting from a smaller to a larger unit requires you to divide. To convert millimetres to metres, the factor is 1000, so you move the decimal point three places to the left.

1.0 2 6

So Seven's height expressed in metres is 1.026m.

Converting from millimetres to centimetres

To convert from millimetres to centimetres, the factor is 10, so you move the decimal point one place to the left.

1 0 2 . 6

So Seven's height expressed in centimetres is 102.6cm.

Converting from centimetres to metres

If you need to express a measurement in centimetres as metres, you will need to divide by 100 (because there are 100cm in 1m).

1 . 0 2 6

102.6cm converts to 1.026m.

Activity 3.5

The patients on Lankie Ward have all had their heights measured. As an exercise, you have been asked to convert their heights as follows.

Express the heights of these patients in centimetres.

1. Oli Dunnitt is 965mm
2. Olivia Stokes is 1.23m
3. Blessed Arwee is 315mm
4. Felicity Farou is 1.09m
5. Morse Elle is 637mm

Convert the units given in the heights of these patients, as indicated.

6. Hank Ittard 0.74m, in cm
7. Marv Illos 0.891m, in cm
8. Brenda Bossie 1.12m, in mm
9. Jenny Aleap 1.09m, in cm
10. Violet Sarblu 1.016m, in mm

Chapter summary

Accurate conversion is an essential skill that every nurse should acquire during their training. This chapter has covered the elements of conversion of metric measures commonly found in healthcare.

In Chapter 5 (Drug calculations) you will see the conversions you have practised here in Chapter 3 put to use when calculating the dosage of medication for patients and service users. You will also come across conversions in Chapter 6 (Calculating intravenous rates) as some intravenous (IV) fluids may require conversion of their units of measurement from litres to millilitres before the rate can be calculated. The amount to be given intravenously must be in millilitres to enable the correct calculation.

Useful websites

Tests and calculations

The following website is useful for metric conversion practice and is free for six months if you register. Try a free download first and register when you need to.

1. Metric conversions quiz

    www.testandcalc.com/quiz/testmet.htm

    These free websites offer guides and resources on metric measure conversions.

BBC Bitesize

2. Measures

    www.bbc.co.uk/schools/ks2bitesize/maths/shape_space/measures/read1.shtml

OpenLearn

3. Numbers, units and arithmetic

    http://labspace.open.ac.uk/course/view.php?id=3434

4. Rounding and estimation

    http://labspace.open.ac.uk/course/view.php?id=3586

Visit the online resources on your computer at **https://study.sagepub.com/starkings krause4e** or on your smart phone or tablet and gain access to:

*   over 400 extra questions to check your learning and gain extra practice;
*   links to useful websites that build on the skills introduced in this chapter;
*   an interactive glossary of key terms.

Answers to the activities

Activity 3.1 (page 42)

Tablets in the Yew Tree Centre ward medicine cabinet are of various strengths per tablet, so each patient will receive their dosage as a combination of the various strengths making up each dosage in the least number of tablets.

1. The strength required is 0.070g.

    0 0 7 0 . 0   So the required amount for Jennie Snoozars is 70mg.

2. The strength required is 0.015g.

    0 0 1 5 . 0   So the required amount for Mitch Crump will be 15mg.

3. The strength required is 0.35g.

0 3 5 0 . 0   So the required amount for Hermany Crusty will be 350mg.

4. The amount required to be converted to mg is 475mcg.

0 . 4 7 5   So the required amount for Walla B will be 0.475mg. Notice that in
                     this conversion the requirement was to divide, therefore the decimal
                     point moved left. Since no decimal point was shown in the original
                     number, the conversion was started from the right-hand end of the
                     number.

5. The amount required to be converted to mg is 0.04g.

0 0 4 0 . 0   So the required amount for Ken Garo will be 40mg.

6. The amount required to be converted to mg is 1750mcg.

1 . 7 5 0   So the required amount for Nickola Surgeon will be 1.75mg. Again in
                     this conversion the requirement was to divide, therefore the decimal
                     point moved left. As no decimal point was shown in the original
                     number, the conversion was started from the right-hand end of the
                     number.

7. The amount required to be converted to mg is 1.02g.

1 0 2 0 . 0   So the required amount for Adi Nahwaz will be 1020mg.

8. The amount required to be converted to mg is 750mcg.

0 . 7 5 0   So the required amount for Andy Ritt will be 0.750mg. Notice
                     that in this conversion the requirement was to divide, therefore
                     the decimal moved left. Since it was not shown in the original
                     number, the conversion was started from the right-hand end
                     of the number.

9. The amount required to be converted to mg is 0.0205g.

0 0 2 0 . 5   So the required amount for Notta Clue will be 20.5mg.

Activity 3.2 (pages 43–4)

1. Justin is under your care and has been ordered 0.095g of penicillin, so the required amount of penicillin in mg is 95mg.

2. Matthew has been prescribed 1.25g/5ml flucloxacillin, so the required amount of flucloxacillin in mg is 250mg/ml.

3. Askme has a mild infection and has been ordered benzyl penicillin from an available mixture of 0.24g/3ml. The amount required in mg is 80mg/ml.

4. Flatulance has been ordered paracetamol, and the stock syrup on hand is 0.35g/7ml, so the required stock strength is 350mg/7ml = 50mg/ml of paracetamol.

Refer back to the ladder and the scenario if you are in any doubt about how to carry out the required conversions.

Activity 3.3 (page 44)

1. Didya Dunnit is prescribed a dose of 0.05g, equal to 50mg.

2. Jose Thisa is prescribed a dose of 0.085g, equal to 85mg.

3. Marie Mevicar is prescribed a dose of 75mcg, equal to 0.075mg.

4. Leif Blowhard is prescribed a dose of 0.17mg, equal to 170mcg.

5. Dunnit Argan is prescribed a dose of 0.705mg, equal to 705mcg.

6. Ruby Rose is prescribed a dose of 0.675mg, equal to 675mcg.

7. Argus Tuft is prescribed a dose of 675mcg, equal to 0.675mg.

8. Wasit Youse is prescribed a dose of 0.035g, equal to 35mg.

9. Well Inever is prescribed a dose of 0.2g, equal to 200mg.

Refer back to the ladder and the scenario if you are in any doubt about how to carry out the required conversions.

Activity 3.4 (pages 45–6)

Convert the patients' weights in grams to kilograms.

1. Digger Hole weighs 61 035g ÷ 1000 = 61.035kg

2. Shaz Ham weighs 5700g ÷ 1000 = 5.7kg

3. Jerry Mander weighs 3247g ÷ 1000 = 3.247kg

4. Alex Uburk weighs 673g ÷ 1000 = 0.673kg

5. Betty Mustgo weighs 1957g ÷ 1000 = 1.957kg

Convert the patients' weights in kilograms to grams.

6. Cerius Lee weighs 2.807kg × 1000 = 2807g

7. Philip Eans weighs 0.108kg × 1000 = 108g

8. Ya Watt weighs 37.63kg × 1000 = 37 630g

9. Ash Ford weighs 24.07kg × 1000 = 24 070g

10. Well Iwood weighs 6.405kg × 1000 = 6405g

Refer back to the ladder and the scenario if you are in any doubt about how to carry out the required conversions.

Activity 3.5 (page 49)

Convert the patients' heights in millimetres or metres to centimetres.

1. Oli Dunnit is 965mm ÷ 10 = 96.5cm

2. Olivia Stokes is 1.23m × 100 = 123cm

3. Blessed Arwee is 315mm ÷ 10 = 31.5cm

4. Felicity Farou is 1.09m × 100 = 109cm

5. Morse Elle is 637mm ÷ 10 = 63.7cm

Convert the patients' heights in metres to the required unit.

6. Hank Ittard 0.74m × 100 = 74cm

7. Marv Illos 0.891m × 100 = 89.1cm

8. Brenda Bossie 1.12m × 1000 = 1120mm

9. Jenny Aleap 1.09m × 100 = 109cm

10. Violet Sarblu 1.016m × 1000 = 1016mm

Refer back to the ladder and the scenario if you are in any doubt about how to carry out the required conversions.

Fluid balance and maintenance

Introduction

The following case study highlights why it is important to make sure fluid balance calculations are correct.

Case study

Mr Matthews is a patient with bronchitis and his doctor is concerned about how much fluid he takes during the day. A nurse is managing his condition and monitoring his fluid balance. Throughout the day the nurse and health care assistant (HCA) keep a record of the fluids consumed by Mr Matthews (such as water, tea, coffee or juice) and all the fluids he excretes (such as urine and vomit). At 12 p.m. the nurse is chatting to the HCA and makes an error in her reading of Mr Matthews' fluid intake. She records that he drank 50ml of water instead of 500ml of water.

Assuming no further errors took place, Mr Matthews' total recorded fluid intake would be 450ml less than he actually consumed. His total fluid balance would therefore be incorrect and the doctor may be further concerned over the amount of fluid Mr Matthews is taking; he could prescribe extra fluid via an intravenous drip which may not otherwise have been prescribed. So it is important that a patient's fluid is collected and recorded correctly; otherwise a patient may be given extra fluid when it is not required, or given medication to excrete more. Correct fluid balance recording enables the best possible decision to be made by healthcare professionals regarding a patient's well-being and recovery schedule.

Errors made in recording fluid intake and output, and incomplete charts, can have serious consequences for the patient. This chapter goes through the essentials required to complete a Fluid Balance Chart accurately.

A Fluid Balance Chart monitors a patient's fluid status and it is an essential requirement for this to be completed accurately. As the case above shows, the consequences of not completing the chart accurately can be serious, and so it is an essential skill that needs to be carried out without errors.

Monitoring fluid balance is an essential aspect of nursing and to be effective it should be accurate, otherwise a patient's condition will be assessed on false information. Fluid intake is usually by oral drinks, food, tube feeds and intravenous fluids. Fluid output usually occurs via urine, vomiting, tube drainage, diarrhoea, sweat, gastric secretions or wound drainage. Accurate measurement of a patient's fluid intake and output will identify those patients at risk of becoming dehydrated (lack of fluid) or overhydrated (too much fluid).

This chapter will help you to understand how to calculate fluid balance and fill out a Fluid Balance Chart correctly. We will first look at what a Fluid Balance Chart is and how to calculate fluid balance. We then show you how to work out fluid intake and fluid output. Finally, we will look at entering, interpreting and calculating data on a Fluid Balance Chart. You should use this in conjunction with other resources and training on how to manage fluids, since this book only covers the numeracy requirements for fluid management.

Fluid Balance Charts and calculating fluid balance

A Fluid Balance Chart measures a patient's hourly fluid intake and output over a 24-hour period. At the end of the 24-hour period the total output (such as urine, drains or other fluid output) is subtracted from the total measured intake (such as oral fluids, intravenous fluids or other inputs). The difference between the input and output is called a fluid balance. It is estimated that an adult person requires between two and a half and three litres of fluid per day.

Fluid balance = Total input − Total output

Scenario

Alan's total intake for a 24-hour period is 1738ml and his total output is 1520ml. You need to find his fluid balance for the 24-hour period.

Alan's fluid balance equals his total intake (or input) of 1738ml minus his total output of 1520ml.

Fluid balance = Total input − Total output
$$= 1738 - 1520$$
$$= 218\text{ml}$$

So the answer is 218ml.

Often the Fluid Balance Chart will not give you the total intake and output but will show you the sums for each intake and output the patient has had. So you need to work out the total intake and output before you can work out the fluid balance.

The scenario below describes what you might face in a practice environment.

Calculating fluid intake

Scenario

Michael Bland had been given the following fluids during a 24-hour period.

Time	Type	Amount
0630	Tea	250ml
0800	Water	200ml
1030	Juice	250ml
1200	Coffee	300ml
1430	Water	300ml
1600	Tea	250ml
1800	Juice	300ml
1930	Water	300ml
2200	Water	300ml

The Ward Sister asks you to calculate Michael Bland's fluid input for the 24-hour period.

To find the total input, add together all the amounts for the 24-hour period. In this case:

Total input = 250 + 200 + 250 + 300 + 300 + 250 + 300 + 300 + 300

        = 2450ml

As you can see, this is an addition calculation, but you need to get this right in order to have the first part of the data needed to calculate the patient's fluid balance.

Calculating fluid output

Scenario

The next part of the data you need is the patient's total output in the 24-hour period. Michael Bland's fluid output during the 24-hour period is measured as follows.

Time	Type	Amount
0600	Urine	300ml
0730	Urine	250ml
0900	Vomit	150ml
1000	Urine	300ml
1130	Urine	210ml
1300	Urine	170ml
1530	Urine	200ml
1730	Urine	250ml
1830	Urine	210ml
2000	Urine	200ml
2200	Urine	150ml

Once again, to find the patient's fluid output for the 24-hour period, add together all the amounts for the 24-hour period. In this case:

Total output = 300 + 250 + 150 + 300 + 210 + 170 + 200 + 250 + 210 + 200 + 150

        = 2390ml

The fluid balance for Michael Bland is found by subtracting the total output from the total input.

Fluid balance = Total input − Total output

        = 2450 − 2390

        = 60ml

In this patient's case the total fluid balance at the end of the 24-hour period is 60ml. Since this is a positive number, it indicates that the patient's intake of fluid is 60ml more than was outputted. However, certain output fluids, such as diarrhoea, are not easy to measure accurately, and it is not possible to measure others, such as sweat. Thus a normal healthy person will appear to have a positive fluid balance. A negative value would indicate that they have excreted more fluid than they have taken in, and that they may become dehydrated.

Now try the following activity to see if you have understood fluid intake and output calculations. You should try the activities without using a calculator.

Activity 4.1

1. Jean Brook had been given the following fluids during a 24-hour period.

Time	Type	Amount
0700	Tea	300ml
0815	Water	150ml
1000	Coffee	300ml
1230	Juice	200ml
1500	Tea	250ml
1620	Tea	250ml
1805	Water	200ml
1910	Coffee	300ml
2130	Water	150ml

What is Jean's fluid input for the 24-hour period?

2. Omar King's fluid output over 24 hours is measured as follows.

Time	Type	Amount
0615	Urine	300ml
0750	Urine	200ml
0910	Urine	170ml
0930	Vomit	130ml
0945	Vomit	100ml
1015	Urine	100ml
1020	Vomit	70ml
1230	Urine	250ml
1515	Urine	200ml
1830	Urine	300ml
2200	Urine	300ml

What is Omar King's output for the 24 hours?

3. Misha Patel's total intake for a 24-hour period is 2110ml and her total output is 1990ml. What is her fluid balance for the 24-hour period?

Answers to all the activities can be found at the end of the chapter.

The next section shows a typical Fluid Balance Chart and will build on the calculations you have done in Activity 4.1.

Reading, interpreting and completing Fluid Balance Charts

The first section of this chapter should have helped you to become competent in calculating fluid inputs, outputs and balances. The following case study shows how a nurse might use these calculations in a practice setting, using a real Fluid Balance Chart. See if you can understand and follow Vera's observations and conclusions.

Case study

Mr Norman Payne has had a heart attack and is on Daffodil Ward in the Woodland Hospital. Close monitoring of his fluid intake and output is required, using a Fluid Balance Chart (FBC), as in Figure 4.1 on page 60.

Vera, the nurse in charge of Mr Payne, examines his chart and from it she observes:

1. the time the FBC commenced;
2. how much had drained from the tube by 1600 hours;
3. what occurred at 1300 hours according to Mr Payne's FBC;
4. Mr Payne's fluid balance at the end of the 24-hour period.

These are her conclusions.

1. The FBC commenced at 0800 hours. The first line started with 250ml of tea under the intake column.
2. By 1600 hours a total of 1200ml had drained from the tube. This is found by adding all the tube drainage, including the 1600 hours line, i.e. 300 + 350 + 200 + 350 = 1200ml.
3. At 1300 hours Mr Payne voided 350ml of urine. This is found by reading across from 1300 to find 350ml in the urine column.
4. Mr Payne's fluid balance at the end of the 24-hour period is 50ml. This is found by subtracting the total output of urine and tube (total output is 1600 + 350 = 1950) from the total input of 2000. Hence 2000 − 1950 = 50ml.

			Clinical Skills Fluid Balance Chart				
Woodland Hospital							
Ward: *Daffodil*			Date: *15/12/17*		M/F: *M*		
Family Name: *Payne*			First Name: *Norman*				
NHS Number: *NA 34 56 78 X*			Date of Birth: *02/09/1932*				

	INTAKE				OUTPUT				
Time	By Mouth or Tube	ml	Intravenous	ml	Urine ml	Vomit or Tube	ml	Other	ml
0100									
0200									
0300									
0400									
0500									
0600									
0700									
0800	*Tea*	*250*							
0900						*Tube*	*300*		
1000	*Coffee*	*300*							
1100						*Tube*	*350*		
1200	*Juice*	*250*							
1300					*350*				
1400	*Tea*	*250*				*Tube*	*200*		
1500									
1600	*Tea*	*250*				*Tube*	*350*		
1700									
1800	*Coffee*	*300*							
1900						*Tube*	*300*		
2000	*Coffee*	*300*							
2100	*Water*	*100*							
2200						*Tube*	*100*		
2300									
2400									
Totals		2000			350		1600		
Total Input		2000			Total Output		1950		
Fluid Balance for time period = 2000 – 1950 = 50ml									

Figure 4.1 Norman Payne's FBC

Now you have seen how a nurse might use a balance chart, attempt using one yourself by completing the following activity.

Activity 4.2

Mrs Janet Rose has pneumonia and is on Bluebell Ward in the Woodland Hospital. Her NHS number is YK 23 17 66 C and her date of birth is 25 May 1950. She requires close monitoring of her fluid intake and output using an FBC.

Mrs Rose was given the following fluids during one 24-hour period.

Time	Type	Amount
0615	Tea	250ml
0730	Water	200ml
0815	Water	200ml
1100	Water	150ml
1230	Juice	200ml
1600	Tea	250ml
1730	Tea	250ml
1930	Water	150ml
2100	Water	200ml

Mrs Rose's fluid output during the same 24-hour period was measured as follows.

Time	Type	Amount
0600	Urine	250ml
0745	Urine	100ml
0800	Vomit	100ml
0900	Urine	150ml
1020	Vomit	100ml
1200	Urine	200ml
1530	Urine	200ml
1700	Urine	250ml
1815	Urine	200ml
2000	Urine	100ml
2130	Urine	100ml

Complete an FBC for her, using the practice FBC at the end of the chapter (page 73), and then answer the following questions:

(Continued)

(Continued)

1. What time did the FBC commence?
2. How much in millilitres did Mrs Rose vomit?
3. What happened between 1200 and 1300 hours according to Mrs Rose's FBC?
4. What is Mrs Rose's fluid balance at the end of the 24-hour period?

Now you have completed a Fluid Balance Chart, you will realise that is important not only that you get the totals and fluid balance correct, but also that you understand what they mean. So take care in your arithmetic and also try to understand the data and what information this is telling you. Is the patient overhydrated or dehydrated? Do you need to raise any concerns to others on the ward?

It may be useful to look at the fluid charts while you are on placement and ask a member of staff to show you how they are completed, as wards or departments do sometimes complete them differently. For example, some fluid charts document 'insensible loss' (sweat) and this has to be included in the calculation. It is also important that you understand what the words on the fluid chart mean so, again, ask if you need help and check if you are unsure.

Case study

Ms Bisi Blanket has been admitted to Daisy Ward in the Woodland Hospital and has an intravenous (IV) drip inserted; 125ml per hour is to be infused. She is not to be given anything orally. Figure 4.2 on page 64 shows her FBC.

Natalie, the nurse in charge of Ms Blanket, examines her chart and from it she observes:

1. the FBC commenced at 0300 hours;
2. by 1600 hours 570ml had drained from the tube;
3. by 1100 hours a total of 1125ml had been infused ('infused' here means 'given'; for example, Ms Blanket has received or been given 1125ml of fluid by a drip);
4. at 1700 hours Ms Blanket voided 200ml of urine;
5. the total amount infused is 2000ml;
6. the total output is 770ml;
7. the fluid balance is 1230ml.

Ms Blanket's fluid output may be considered quite low at the moment so you may need to keep monitoring her fluid balance for another 24-hour period, especially considering she has been on an IV drip. Intravenous drip rates will be covered in Chapter 6.

Activity 4.3

Look at Ms Sarah Gore's FBC, shown in Figure 4.3 on page 65, and answer the following questions.

1. At what time did Ms Gore's FBC commence?

    a. 0500 hours
    b. 0400 hours
    c. 1600 hours

2. What occurred at 1700 hours, according to Ms Gore's FBC?

    a. Ms Gore voided 150ml of urine
    b. Ms Gore was given 150ml of fluid orally
    c. Ms Gore voided 200ml of urine

3. How much was drained by tube by 1200 hours?

    a. 400ml
    b. 250ml
    c. 150ml

4. How much IV fluid had Ms Gore had up to 1400 hours?

    a. 125ml
    b. 550ml
    c. 1250ml
    d. 800ml

5. What was Ms Gore's fluid balance?

    a. 1350ml
    b. −750ml
    c. −100ml
    d. 1250ml

Did you find some of these activities more difficult than others? Did you notice, for example, that the question in part 3 of Activity 4.3 was asking how much was drained by tube, not how much was outputted altogether by 1200 hours? You need to take care to understand what is being asked, or what information you need to find out, and ensure you read the chart correctly and find the appropriate data before beginning the calculation. This skill is essential for a registered nurse and will be important from the very start of your practice placements.

Woodland Hospital	Clinical Skills Fluid Balance Chart	
Ward: *Daisy*	Date: *11/12/17*	M/F: *F*
Family Name: *Blanket*	First Name: *Bisi*	
NHS Number: *XY 45 67 89 A*	Date of Birth: *02/12/1970*	

	INTAKE				OUTPUT				
Time	By Mouth or Tube	ml	Intravenous	ml	Urine ml	Vomit or Tube	ml	Other	ml
0100									
0200									
0300	*Nil orally*		*Saline*	125					
0400				125					
0500				125					
0600				125					
0700				125		*Tube*	200		
0800				125					
0900				125					
1000				125					
1100				125					
1200				125		*Tube*	180		
1300				125					
1400				125					
1500				125					
1600				125		*Tube*	190		
1700				125	200				
1800				125					
1900									
2000									
2100									
2200									
2300									
2400									
Totals				2000	200		570		
Total Input				2000	Total Output		770		
Fluid Balance for time period = 2000 − 770 = 1230ml									

Figure 4.2   Bisi Blanket's FBC

Woodland Hospital	Clinical Skills Fluid Balance Chart	
Ward: *Tulip*	Date: *12/12/2017*	M/F: *F*
Family Name: *Gore*	First Name: *Sarah*	
NHS Number: *YB 78 12 34 B*	Date of Birth: *21/03/1970*	

	INTAKE				OUTPUT				
Time	By Mouth or Tube	ml	Intravenous	ml	Urine ml	Vomit or Tube	ml	Other	ml
0100									
0200									
0300									
0400	*Nil by Mouth*		*Saline*	125					
0500				125	*100*				
0600				125		*Tube*	250		
0700				125					
0800				125	*100*				
0900				125					
1000				125		*Tube*	150		
1100				125	*100*				
1200				125					
1300				125					
1400					*150*	*Tube*	130		
1500									
1600									
1700					*200*				
1800						*Tube*	220		
1900									
2000									
2100					*300*				
2200						*Tube*	300		
2300									
2400									
Totals				1250	950		1050		
Total Input				1250	Total Output		2000		
Fluid Balance for time period = 1250 – 2000 = –750ml									

Figure 4.3 Sarah Gore's FBC

Children's fluid balance

Children's fluid balance is calculated in the same way as the adult ones you have been looking at. The major difference is that a child's fluid intake and output will usually be much lower than that of an adult. You will also have to calculate, particularly for very young children, how much urine has been outputted from a wet nappy.

Scenario

Omar Hassan is six weeks old and has been admitted to hospital. He has a wet nappy. The nappy weighed 15g when dry, and his nappy now weighs 127g. You need to find how much urine Omar has passed.

To find how much urine Omar has passed, you need to subtract the weight of the dry nappy from the weight of the wet nappy. You need to remember 1g = 1ml. So the amount of urine passed in this case is 127 − 15 = 112 ml.

The 112ml is then added under the urine column of Omar's Fluid Balance Chart at the time you weighed the nappy and will be used to calculate his total fluid output and, in turn, his fluid balance.

Activity 4.4

Gloria Parker is ten weeks old and has been admitted to hospital. She has a wet nappy. The nappy weighed 18g when dry, and her nappy now weighs 132g. How much urine did Gloria pass since her last nappy change?

Case study

Miss Amber Brown has been admitted to Buttercup Ward in the Woodland Hospital with respiratory problems. She has been put on close monitoring of her fluid intake and output using an FBC (see Figure 4.4 on page 67).

Julie, the nurse looking after Amber, has found that a nappy change at 2300 hours was not recorded. Her fluid balance will now have to be altered to include the urine passed at this time. Her dry nappy would have weighed 25g. Her wet nappy weighed 164g.

		Clinical Skills Fluid Balance Chart		
Woodland Hospital				
Ward: *Buttercup*		Date: *02/05/17*		M/F: *F*
Family Name: *Brown*		First Name: *Amber*		
NHS Number: *654321*		Date of Birth: *21/01/2010*		

	INTAKE				OUTPUT				
Time	By Mouth or Tube	ml	Intravenous	ml	Urine ml	Vomit or Tube	ml	Other	ml
0100									
0200									
0300									
0400									
0500									
0600	Milk	150			155				
0700									
0800									
0900									
1000	Milk	127			143				
1100									
1200					125				
1300									
1400	Milk	172			100				
1500									
1600									
1700									
1800	Milk	125			154				
1900									
2000									
2100					60				
2200	Milk	175							
2300									
2400									
Totals	749				737				
Total Input	749				Total Output		737		
Fluid Balance for time period = 749 – 737 = 12ml									

Figure 4.4 Amber Brown's FBC

First we calculate the amount of urine passed: 164 − 25 = 139ml. This amount is then added to her fluid output giving a total fluid output of 737 + 139 = 876ml. Her fluid balance will now be 749 − 876 = −127ml. This value indicates that she has excreted more fluid than she has taken in over this time period. Since this is a negative value it would be wise to pass this information on to the health official in charge of Amber's case.

Figure 4.4 is an example of a child's Fluid Balance Chart. Now have a go at the following activity.

Activity 4.5

Omar Mohamed has been admitted to Buttercup Ward in the Woodland Hospital with suspected meningitis. He has been put on close monitoring of his fluid intake and output using an FBC. All dry nappies for Omar weigh 20g. His NHS number is NB 271546X and his date of birth is 30 June 2017. Complete an FBC for him, using the practice chart at the end of the chapter.

1. Omar's nappy was changed at the following times:

Time	Weight (g)
0600	152
0730	140
1200	125
1415	100
1730	160

Add the amount of urine passed to Omar's FBC.

2. Omar was given feeds of infant milk:

Time	Amount (ml)
0630	150
0800	100
1130	130
1700	150
2115	120

Add these to Omar's FBC.

3. Now work out Omar's fluid balance.

Chapter summary

Accurate recording of fluid intake and output is a requirement for nurses. Do remember to measure all fluid intake and output and record the amount, along with the type of fluid. If you delegate the task, make sure you get the correct totals. For example, if a patient is able they could record their own intake and output using appropriate measuring devices. Measure all fluids, as far as possible, in a calibrated container so that measures are accurate. Update the Fluid Balance Chart on a regular basis. The fluid balance for a 24-hour period is calculated by using the following formula:

Fluid balance = Total input − Total output

Useful websites

The following websites offer revision material that you can use to enhance your numeracy skills. The pages listed below are accessible free of charge and can be used to help you with the arithmetic required for this chapter.

BBC Bitesize

1. Addition

    www.bbc.co.uk/schools/ks2bitesize/maths/number/addition/read1.shtml

2. Subtraction

    www.bbc.co.uk/schools/ks2bitesize/maths/number/subtraction/read1.shtml

3. Rules of arithmetic

    www.bbc.co.uk/education/topics/znmtsbk

Visit the online resources on your computer at **https://study.sagepub.com/ starkingskrause4e** or on your smart phone or tablet and gain access to:

- over 400 extra questions to check your learning and gain extra practice;
- links to useful websites that build on the skills introduced in this chapter;
- an interactive glossary of key terms.

Answers to the activities

Activity 4.1 (pages 58–9)

1. Total input = 300 + 150 + 300 + 200 + 250 + 250 + 200 + 300 + 150 = 2100ml
2. Total output = 300 + 200 + 170 + 130 + 100 + 100 + 70 + 250 + 200 + 300 + 300 = 2120ml
3. Fluid balance = Total input − Total output

    $$= 2110 − 1990$$

    $$= 120ml$$

If you got the arithmetic incorrect here you may wish to refer to Chapter 2 on addition and subtraction, and/or look at web pages 1, 2 and 3, listed above, for further practice.

Activity 4.2 (pages 61–2)

The FBC on page 71 shows how you should have filled in the chart.

1. The Fluid Balance Chart commenced at 0600 hours.
2. Mrs Rose vomited 100ml at 0800 hours and 100ml at 1020 hours. Her total vomit is therefore 100 + 100 = 200ml.
3. Mrs Rose voided 200ml of urine at 1200 hours and at 1230 hours she had 200ml of juice.
4. Mrs Woodstock's fluid balance is 100ml.

Activity 4.3 (page 63)

1. b
2. c
3. a
4. c
5. b

Activity 4.4 (page 66)

The amount of urine passed by Gloria is 132 − 18 = 114ml.

The 114ml is then added under the urine column of Gloria's FBC at the time you weighed the nappy and will be used to calculate her total fluid output and, in turn, her fluid balance.

Activity 4.5 (page 68)

The FBC on page 72 shows how you should have filled in the chart.

Remember to take off the weight of the dry nappy, in this case 20g, from the weight of the wet nappy to get the correct urine total. The amount of urine at 0600 hours is then 152 − 20 = 132ml. The correct urine totals to be placed on the FBC are as follows:

Time	Wet weight (g)	Urine (ml)
0600	152	132
0730	140	120
1200	125	105
1415	100	80
1730	160	140

Fluid balance = Total input − Total output
= 650 − 577
= 73ml

Omar's fluid balance is 73ml

Woodland Hospital	Clinical Skills Fluid Balance Chart	
Ward: *Bluebell*	Date: *12/11/17*	M/F: *F*
Family Name: *Rose*	First Name: *Janet*	
NHS Number: *YK 23 17 66 C*	Date of Birth: *25/05/1950*	

	INTAKE				OUTPUT				
Time	By Mouth or Tube	ml	Intravenous	ml	Urine ml	Vomit or Tube	ml	Other	ml
0100									
0200									
0300									
0400									
0500									
0600	Tea	250			250				
0700	Water	200			100				
0800	Water	200				Vomit	100		
0900					150				
1000						Vomit	100		
1100	Water	150							
1200	Juice	200			200				
1300									
1400									
1500					200				
1600	Tea	250							
1700	Tea	250			250				
1800					200				
1900	Water	150							
2000					100				
2100	Water	200			100				
2200									
2300									
2400									
Totals		1850			1550		200		
Total Input		1850			**Total Output**		1750		
Fluid Balance for time period = 1850 – 1750 = 100ml									

Figure 4.5 Janet Rose's FBC

Woodland Hospital	Clinical Skills Fluid Balance Chart	
Ward: *Buttercup*	Date: *01/11/2017*	M/F: *M*
Family Name: *Mohamed*	First Name: *Omar*	
NHS Number: *NB 271546 X*	Date of Birth: *30/06/2017*	

	INTAKE				OUTPUT					
Time	By Mouth or Tube	ml	Intravenous	ml	Urine ml	Vomit or Tube	ml	Other	ml
0100									
0200									
0300									
0400									
0500									
0600	*Milk*	*150*			*132*				
0700					*120*				
0800	*Milk*	*100*							
0900									
1000									
1100	*Milk*	*130*							
1200					*105*				
1300									
1400					*80*				
1500									
1600									
1700	*Milk*	*150*			*140*				
1800									
1900									
2000									
2100	*Milk*	*120*							
2200									
2300									
2400									
Totals		*650*			*577*				
Total Input		*650*			Total Output		*577*		
Fluid Balance for time period = 650 – 577 = 73ml									

Figure 4.6   Omar Mohamed's FBC

Appendix

Sample FBC

Woodland Hospital	Clinical Skills Fluid Balance Chart
Ward:	Date: M/F:
Family Name:	First Name:
NHS Number:	Date of Birth:

| Time | INTAKE | | | | OUTPUT | | | | |
	By Mouth or Tube	ml	Intravenous	ml	Urine ml	Vomit or Tube	ml	Other	ml
0100									
0200									
0300									
0400									
0500									
0600									
0700									
0800									
0900									
1000									
1100									
1200									
1300									
1400									
1500									
1600									
1700									
1800									
1900									
2000									
2100									
2200									
2300									
2400									
Totals									
Total Input					Total Output				

Chapter 5 Drug calculations

Chapter aims

By the end of this chapter you should be able to:

- calculate the number of tablets required for patients from their prescription;
- calculate the dose required in liquid form as prescribed;
- calculate the drug dose for injection;
- calculate the drug dose for injection for patients requiring insulin;
- work out the dose to be given to a patient when prescribed by body weight.

Introduction

The following case study highlights why it is important to make sure drug calculations are correct.

Case study

Bex's nursing duties include giving the pre-medication for patients about to have surgery in the operating theatre; this relaxes the patient before they are wheeled down to the theatre. The anaesthetist can then place an endotracheal tube into the patient's trachea in order to ensure that the airway is not closed off and that air can reach the lungs during surgery.

An inexperienced doctor drew up what he thought was the correct pre-medication dose for one of Bex's patients, but made a mistake in the volume required and under-estimated the dose. The result was that the patient was not sufficiently relaxed and was extremely uncomfortable when the endotracheal tube was inserted.

The endotracheal tube can be inserted in an emergency without the aid of any relaxation but this is extremely uncomfortable and generally to be avoided in other circumstances.

In some cases the anaesthetist is unable to insert the endotracheal tube and surgery has to be postponed, causing distress to patients and disturbance to schedules.

Correct calculations are essential for all concerned.

This chapter covers a variety of numerical and mathematical tasks which nurses may be required to perform in practice.

This book does not cover reconstitution of a powder drug. Drugs are mainly stored in powder form because they are often unstable in liquid form and are only made up into a solution just before use. Consult the pharmacist at your place of work for help in reconstitution of solutions.

During your nursing career you will administer and later supervise the administration of all types of medicines. To do this safely the development of certain numerical and mathematical skills, as seen in Chapter 2, is essential. Your calculations must be accurate in order to ensure that the safety of patients is not compromised.

During your course your ability in drug calculations will be examined, usually by a series of tests which help you develop your skills and which are done without the use of a calculator. This is to check that you have mastered the **Essential Skills Clusters** 33(i) and 33(ii). It is suggested that you practise the calculations in this chapter without using a calculator. If your training institution allows you to use one then by all means do so, but be aware that some assessments may need to be completed without using a calculator.

Many nurses have difficulty with drug calculations, usually because they are not confident with the numeracy and mathematics required. Practising drug calculations will help you develop these skills and become more confident with the calculations needed. Checking colleagues' calculations is another way to check your understanding of the numerical concepts involved in drug calculations.

Many drugs require some type of calculation prior to administration, and before you start this chapter you will need to be able to convert from one metric unit to another. Chapter 3 has examples of this skill and can be used for revision if necessary. Table 5.1 is a reminder of the types of conversions with which you will need to be familiar.

Unit	Abbreviation	Equivalent	Abbreviation
1 kilogram	kg	1000 grams	g
1 gram	g	1000 milligrams	mg
1 milligram	mg	1000 micrograms	mcg
1 microgram	mcg	1000 nanograms	ng
1 litre	l	1000 millilitres	ml

Table 5.1 Equivalents of common units of measurement

Notice that the abbreviation for litres is the small letter 'l': be careful not to confuse this with the numeral 1.

How drugs are administered

There are three main ways that drugs can be administered:

- **orally** (by mouth);
- by **injection**;
- or by **intravenous infusion**.

This chapter will look at drugs given orally by tablets or in liquid form and by injection. Intravenous (IV) infusion will be covered in Chapter 6. You will need to apply previous knowledge in order to complete this chapter so look back, particularly at Chapters 2 and 3, and revise when you need to.

Calculating a dose involving tablets

Drugs may be administered in many ways; a common means is orally, in the form of tablets. Whole tablets are always preferable to broken tablets; never use less than half a tablet for a patient. Broken tablets are harder to identify as many tablets look the same and a patient could be given the wrong tablet, which will not help their recovery progress. If a tablet has been broken in half always use the 'other' half for the next dose for the same patient, making sure you keep the broken tablet in the correctly labelled container. Tablets are often marked with the weight of drug which they contain.

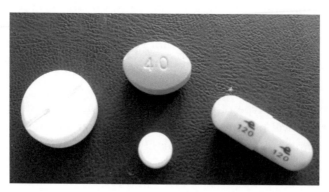

Figure 5.1   Oral medications

As with any calculation involving the administration of drugs, it is absolutely vital that the same unit of weight is used throughout the calculation. Weight is the amount of drug contained in the tablet. Always check that both the **prescribed strength** (**strength required** by the patient) and the **stock strength/dispensed dose** (the weight of tablet in the medicine cabinet) are in the same units. For example, both could be in milligrams (mg), or both in micrograms (mcg).

Often one of the units needs to be converted and this must be done before any calculation is started (Chapter 3 covers conversion rates). This ensures that the patient gets the correct dose. For example, if the prescribed dose is in milligrams and the tablets are in micrograms, ignoring the units would mean that the patient could be given an incorrect dose. An incorrect calculation of this sort can seriously harm a patient's recovery or indeed cause further illness.

It is safer, and therefore best practice, to convert to the lowest level of unit. Once the strength required and stock strength are both in the same units, we can calculate the number of tablets required.

The method for calculating the number of tablets is the same for all drug doses, and uses this formula:

$$\frac{\text{Strength required}}{\text{Stock strength}} \times \text{Volume of stock solution}$$

Since we are dealing with tablets here, the volume of the stock solution will always be one tablet. Therefore the formula for calculating how many tablets a patient should receive is:

$$\frac{\text{Strength required}}{\text{Stock strength}} \times \text{One tablet}$$

Since tablets are never broken to less than half a tablet, the answer should always be half a tablet, a whole number of tablets, or a whole number plus half a tablet. However, bear in mind that if the tablet is not scored (with a groove down the middle) it must not be broken and the dose given must be to the nearest tablet.

Check with the patient's consultant and/or pharmacist if you have any concern about the dose. For example, if you think the dose is too high or low for the patient, then it is always best to check.

You may find it helpful to use this mnemonic:

N = Need (the strength required/prescribed strength)

H = Have (what you have as stock strength)

S = Stock (volume of stock strength)

And the formula in this case would be:

$$\frac{N}{H} \times \frac{S}{1} = \text{The correct dose for the patient}$$

The numeral 1 under the 'S' is there to prevent you making mistakes during your calculations.

Scenario

Linda Orchid suffers from epilepsy and has been ordered 45mg of phenobarbitone to be given orally. Stock on hand is 30mg tablets. You need to find the number of tablets required for Linda.

To find out how many tablets Linda requires, you need to abstract the relevant pieces of information. The strength required here is 45mg and the stock strength is 30mg. Using the formula above and inserting the relevant values we do the calculation:

$$\frac{\text{Strength required}}{\text{Stock strength}} \times \text{One tablet}$$

$$\frac{45}{30} \times 1 = 1\frac{1}{2} \text{ tablets}$$

Or, using the NHS mnemonic where you Need 45mg, you Have 30mg, and the Stock is one tablet:

$$\frac{N}{H} \times \frac{S}{1} = \text{The correct dose for the patient}$$

$$\frac{45}{30} \times 1 = 1\frac{1}{2} \text{ tablets}$$

So Linda needs to take $1\frac{1}{2}$ tablets to get 45mg of phenobarbitone as prescribed. (Please note although this example has half a tablet for illustrative purposes, you should check in your own practice whether breaking a tablet is allowable.)

Notice that both the stock strength and the strength required are in milligrams, so no conversion between units is necessary. The next scenario is one where a conversion has to take place before the formula can be used.

Scenario

Bailey Beetle has heart problems and has been ordered 0.25mg of digoxin to be given orally. Stock on hand is 125mcg tablets. You need to find the number of tablets that Bailey should be given.

Notice that the stock required (what you need) is in milligrams (mg) and the stock strength (what you have) is in micrograms (mcg). First you need to convert these both to the same units. Using Table 5.1 we can see that to get 0.25mg into micrograms we move the decimal point (equivalent to multiplying by 1000) three places to the right as follows:

0.25mg = 250mcg

Now both stock strength (Have) and strength required (Need) are in the same units and we can use the formula above to put in the numerical values.

$$\frac{\text{Strength required}}{\text{Stock strength}} \times \text{One tablet}$$

$$\frac{250}{125} \times 1 = 2\,\text{tablets}$$

Or, using the NHS mnemonic where you Need 250mg, you Have 125mg, and the Stock is one tablet we have:

$$\frac{N}{H} \times \frac{S}{1} = \text{The correct dose for the patient}$$

$$\frac{250}{125} \times 1 = 2\,\text{tablets}$$

So Bailey needs to have two tablets of digoxin from the stock cupboard to get the correct dose as ordered.

Now try the following activity to see if you have understood how to use the formula to calculate how many tablets the patients require. Remember that you may need to do a conversion so that both stock strength (what you have) and stock required (what you need) are in the same units. You should try the activities without using a calculator.

Activity 5.1

Warfarin is an anticoagulant and helps to prevent clots in veins, arteries, lungs or heart. Warfarin comes in tablet form; the tablets that are kept in the medicine cabinet are of stock strength 5mg; they are scored. The following residents at Garden View Care Home are being treated with this drug and will be taking the tablet(s) once a day. Calculate the number of tablets required for the following patients.

1. Jim Bow needs to have 2500mcg
2. Jess Rarebit needs to have 7.5mg
3. Alf Ensafety needs to have 0.005g

(Continued)

(Continued)

Prazosin is an antihypertensive drug which works by relaxing the blood vessels. The stock strength of the tablets kept in the medicine cabinet is 2mg per tablet; the tablets are scored. The following patients with high blood pressure are being treated with this drug once a day. Calculate the number required for the following patients.

4. Pur Feck needs to have 0.005g
5. Fan Tessie needs to have 2000mcg
6. Fatma Dyet needs to have 5mg

Thioridazine is in a class of drugs called phenothiazines. The drug works by changing the actions of chemicals in the brain and is typically used for psychotic disorders, such as schizophrenia. Thioridazine is generally reserved for people who do not respond to other drugs or who cannot take other drugs because of their side effects. The strength of stock kept in the medicine cabinet is 50mg per tablet; the tablets are scored. The following patients are being treated with this drug in one daily dose. Calculate the number of tablets required for the following patients.

7. James Glu needs to have 0.075g
8. Uri Kiddin needs to have 25mg
9. Noah Way needs to have 0.15g

Answers to all the activities can be found at the end of the chapter.

The questions in Activity 5.1 refer to tablets and not capsules. If drugs are in capsule form, then you must not open or split them. Doses are calculated to the nearest whole capsule. Should you have any queries, consult the person in charge at your place of work and/or the pharmacist or doctor who prescribed the drug.

Some drugs come in various forms such as mixtures, capsules or even powder, which is mixed with water before the drug is given. You must take great care when reading the prescribed order regarding in what form the drug is to be given. The next section will look at drugs in liquid form.

Calculating a dose involving mixtures

Drugs are often stocked in the form of suspensions, syrup or mixtures. Before measuring out any of these mixtures you should thoroughly shake the container so that the drug is evenly mixed, otherwise the incorrect dose may be given.

Having ensured that the mixture is thoroughly mixed, you can measure the prescribed dose. To calculate the amount required, use the same method as for all drug calculations, with this formula:

$$\frac{\text{Strength required}}{\text{Stock strength}} \times \text{Volume of stock solution}$$

Alternatively, use the NHS mnemonic:

$$\frac{N}{H} \times \frac{S}{1} = \text{The correct dose for the patient}$$

Scenario

Cyril Michaels, from Rosela Children's Home, has been ordered three doses of 500mg of penicillin per day to treat his bacterial infection; stock mixture on hand is syrup 125mg/5ml. You need to work out what volume of syrup per dose should be given to Cyril, and his total daily dose.

To find out how many millilitres Cyril requires you need to abstract the relevant pieces of information. The strength or amount required is 500mg and the stock strength is 125mg/5ml. The 125mg/5ml means that there is 125mg of drug per 5ml of mixture.

Using the formula or NHS mnemonic above gives the following calculation:

The volume required, in ml, is $\dfrac{500}{125} \times \dfrac{5}{1}$

First you cancel down, as shown in Chapter 2. Cancel by 125, since 125 goes once into 125 and four times into 500, giving:

$$\frac{4}{1} \times \frac{5}{1} = 4 \times 5 = 20\text{ml}$$

So Cyril needs 20ml of the mixture to receive 500mg of penicillin as prescribed per dose. His total dose for the day (he is to be given three doses) is then found by multiplying the dose by three, that is, $20 \times 3 = 60\text{ml}$.

This prescription has both the stock strength and the strength required in milligrams so no conversion was required. The next scenario is one where a conversion has to take place before the formula can be used.

Notice here that the units are different; one is in grams and the other is in milligrams. You need to convert the prescribed dose to milligrams before you use the formula. Refer to Table 5.1 on page 75 for conversion rates. In this case 0.4g = 400mg (you move the decimal point three places to the right).

Scenario

Leonard, a patient on Saffron Ward, has been ordered flucloxacillin 0.4g orally to treat his chest infection; stock syrup on hand is 125mg/5ml. You need to work out what volume of syrup should be given to Leonard.

The strength or amount required is 400mg and the stock strength is 125mg/5ml. Using the formula or NHS mnemonic given above gives the following calculation:

The volume required, in ml, is $\dfrac{400}{125} \times \dfrac{5}{1}$

First you cancel down, as shown in Chapter 2. Cancel by 25, since 25 goes 5 times into 125 and 16 times into 400, giving:

$$\dfrac{16}{5} \times \dfrac{5}{1}$$

You can then cancel out the 5s to give 16ml. So Leonard needs 16ml of the mixture to receive 400mg of flucloxacillin as prescribed.

Whether the drug is in the form of a syrup or in a suspension, the calculation remains the same; in both cases, always shake the container to ensure a proper distribution of the drug before measuring.

Remember, before doing any calculations make sure that the strength required and stock strength are in the same units. As a general rule of thumb, always convert to the smaller unit; for example, if you are dealing with both grams and milligrams, it is better to work in milligrams, as in the scenario with Leonard above.

You should try the following activity without using a calculator.

Activity 5.2

1. Jill from Rosehip Respite Centre has been ordered 1.5g orally of penicillin for her throat infection; stock syrup on hand is 250mg/ml. What volume of syrup is required for her dose?
2. Patrick, an in-patient at the Eagle View Mental Health Respite Lodge, has a severe chest infection and has been prescribed 750mg flucloxacillin orally; stock suspension on hand is 500mg/2ml. How much stock suspension is required per dose for him? He is to have four doses per day. How much flucloxacillin does he receive in one day?

3. Amelia has a wound infection after her operation and has been ordered benzyl penicillin 600mg orally; stock mixture on hand is 150mg/2.5ml. Calculate the volume of mixture to be given to Amelia.

4. Tawdry has been ordered paracetamol 625mg three times a day orally to help ease her pain after having her wisdom teeth out; stock syrup on hand is 125mg/1.5ml. What volume of syrup should be given to Tawdry per dose? How much paracetamol does she receive per day?

So far we have looked at drugs that have been given orally. The next two sections will look at drugs that are administered by injection.

Calculating a drug dose for injection

The previous section looked at drugs in liquid form that were given orally; another way of administering drugs in liquid form is by injection. When calculating a dose to be given by injection the number of decimal places used in the calculations should match the graduations on the syringe that you are going to use (see Figures 5.3 and 5.4 below).

Notice that, unlike tablets where the dose is calculated in whole and half numbers, liquids to be given by injection can be measured in a narrower range.

As with any calculation involving the administration of drugs, it is absolutely vital that the same unit of capacity is used throughout the calculation. Always check that both strength required and stock strength are in the same unit. The most common is to have both in grams (g), both in milligrams (mg) or both in micrograms (mcg). Any conversion must be done before the dosage calculation is started. See Chapter 3 for revision on conversions.

The volume that the liquid is prepared in must also be noted, because the result of the calculation will be an amount in this unit of measure. For example, if the drug comes in milligrams per millilitre the required dose will be calculated and drawn up in millilitres (ml). In the case of insulin, which comes in units, then the dose would be drawn up in units.

Once the strength required and stock strength are both in the same units of measurement, you can begin to calculate the amount of stock solution required. The formula for calculating liquid drug doses is the same as for those we have already done:

$$\frac{\text{Strength required}}{\text{Stock strength}} \times \text{Volume of stock solution}$$

Alternatively, use the NHS mnemonic:

$$\frac{N}{H} \times \frac{S}{1} = \text{The correct dose for the patient}$$

As well as calculating the correct volume of drug to be given, you also need to select the correct syringe (see Figure 5.2) to use and draw up the volume required. Typical sizes of syringes used for injections in hospitals and clinics in the UK are 1ml, 2ml, 3ml, 5ml, 10ml, 20ml, 30ml and 50ml.

For example, if you need to draw up 0.8ml then you would use a 1ml syringe (see Figure 5.3). To draw up 3ml you would use a slightly larger syringe (see Figure 5.4).

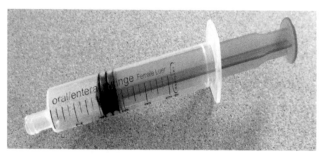

Figure 5.2   A typical syringe

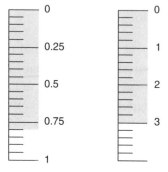

Figure 5.3   *Figure 5.4*

So first work out, using the formula, how much drug in volume you need to administer; then select the correct syringe size; and finally draw up the volume required.

Scenario

Scopolamine, an anticholinergic medicine, is being used to ease Mrs Vera Bland's nausea as she recovers from surgery. She has been ordered 0.25mg of scopolamine. Stock on hand is 0.4mg/2ml. You need to work out how much is to be drawn up for her dose.

To find out how much is to be drawn up for Vera's injection you need to abstract the relevant pieces of information. Notice that the amount prescribed and the stock on hand are both in decimal form. It is easier if you convert both amounts to micrograms; using the conversion Table 5.1 you have:

0.25mg = 250mcg

0.4mg = 400mcg

The strength required (Need) is 250mcg.

The stock strength (Have) is 400mcg.

The volume of stock solution (Stock) is 2ml.

Using the formula given above gives the following calculation:

$$\frac{\text{Strength required}}{\text{Stock strength}} \times \text{Volume of stock solution}$$

Alternatively, use the NHS mnemonic:

$$\frac{N}{H} \times \frac{S}{1} = \text{The correct dose for the patient}$$

$$\frac{250}{400} \times \frac{2}{1} = 1.25\text{ml}$$

So you need to select a 2ml syringe to draw up the 1.25ml required for Vera's injection (see Figure 5.5).

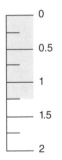

Figure 5.5

A common error made here is to just ignore (or misread due to haste) the decimal points. This would result in the following calculation:

$$\frac{25}{4} \times \frac{2}{1} = 12.5\text{ml}, \textit{ which is (VERY) incorrect and potentially lethal.}$$

This would result in a huge overdose for the patient, as well as a large volume to be injected. Now try the following activity and see if you can work out how much drug to draw up and what syringe size to use.

Activity 5.3

Morphine is in a group of drugs called narcotic pain relievers. It is used to treat moderate to severe pain. The following patients in Serenity Hospice have cancer and have been prescribed morphine to ease their pain.

Morphine of stock strength 15mg/ml is in the medicine cabinet. Calculate the amount to be drawn up and the syringe size to use for injection for the following patients.

1. Harpa Severn is prescribed a dose of 0.15g
2. Happie Agen is prescribed a dose of 6mg
3. Whats Ittoya is prescribed a dose of 22.5mg

Pethidine is a painkilling drug used to ease pain during labour. The following patients have been prescribed a single dose of pethidine.

The stock strength of pethidine in the medicine cabinet is 100mg/2ml. Calculate the amount to be drawn up and the syringe size to use for injection for the following patients.

4. Janice Poplin is prescribed a dose of 0.3g
5. Pep Ermint is prescribed a dose of 65mg
6. Crystal Stone is prescribed a dose of 87mg

Cortisone is a powerful anti-inflammatory medication. The following residents in Sunland Farm Care Home have arthritis and have been prescribed cortisone to ease their inflammatory pain.

Cortisone of stock strength 125mg/5ml is in the medicine cabinet. Calculate the amount to be drawn up and the syringe size to use for injection for the following patients.

7. Bren Gunna is prescribed a dose of 0.06g
8. Hugh Lorrie is prescribed a dose of 150mg
9. Kiera Nowt is prescribed a dose of 75mg

The next section will look at giving injections of insulin.

Calculating a drug dose by injection for insulin doses

The strength of insulin is measured by the number of insulin units contained in 1ml. For example U.10 or 10U means that there are 10 units of insulin per millilitre. A 1ml syringe would normally be used. This syringe is graduated in tenths of a millilitre.

Syringes are usually graduated in units for the type of insulin prescribed so make sure you use the correct syringe or you will have to adjust the volume required. Insulin keeps blood glucose levels under control for people with diabetes, and is prescribed in terms of units.

Scenario

Jonathon Paul has U.40 insulin and needs to have a dose of 28 units. You have a syringe graduated to be used with U.40 insulin. You need to work out how much is to be drawn up for him using the U.40 insulin.

U.40 means that there are 40 units contained in one millilitre. You need to find the amount to draw up into the syringe so that Jonathon gets a dose of 28 units. This is a fraction problem; you need to find what proportion 28 units is of 40 units. This can be expressed as a fraction:

$$\frac{28}{40} = 0.7\text{ml}$$

Jonathon is to have 0.7ml of insulin drawn up for his injection.

Fractions were covered in Chapter 2 so look back if you need to revise here. Now try the following activity to test your understanding of insulin doses.

Activity 5.4

1. Two patients newly diagnosed with diabetes at the Diabetes Clinic require insulin injections.

Name	Dose to be given	Strength of solution
Pauline Booker	60 units	U.20
Maj Ick	30 units	U.40

    How much insulin is to be drawn up for these patients using the strengths given?

2. A syringe is graduated in units for use with U.40 insulin. To what graduation mark should it be filled to give a dose of 32 units, if only U.20 insulin is available?

We now look at drugs that are prescribed by body weight.

Drug dose by body weight

At times drug doses may be ordered based on a patient's body weight, especially with children's doses (see Chapter 7). When calculating body weight doses you need to make sure that all measurements are in the same units before working out the dose required. For revision on conversions see Chapter 3.

Drugs will usually be ordered in milligrams per kilogram of body weight per day, divided up into a number of doses per day. So first of all calculate the total dose for the day for the patient and then divide up this total into the number of doses per day. Remember that you always need to calculate the single dose rate to administer the correct dose each time.

Scenario

Austen Major has been prescribed erythromycin. The dose prescribed is 50mg/kg/day, four doses daily. Austen was weighed today, in the care home, and his weight is 84kg. You need to find what total dose Austen requires and then calculate the single dose to be given to him.

To find out how much Austen requires you need to abstract the relevant pieces of information. The dose 50mg/kg/day means that for every kilogram Austen weighs he needs 50mg of erythromycin; Austen weighs 84kg. So the total daily requirement for Austen is $84 \times 50 = 4200$mg. Austen is to be given four doses a day, so you need to divide the 4200mg into four equal doses.

$4200 \div 4 = 1050$mg per dose.

Austen needs each dose to be of 1050mg.

Now try the following activity regarding dose by body weight. Children's doses will be covered in Chapter 7.

Activity 5.5

Chloramphenicol is given to patients, particularly after an operation, to help treat infection. The following patients on your ward have been ordered chloramphenicol by their body weight. Calculate the total dose prescribed and how much each dose in grams is to be for the following patients.

1. Ben Daguy weighs 55kg and is prescribed 20mg/kg/day to be given in four doses.
2. Jens Mellie weighs 64kg and is prescribed 100mg/kg/day divided into doses to be given every 6 hours for the next 24 hours.
3. Okao Fornow weighs 72kg and is prescribed 50mg/kg/day in four equal doses.

Calculating drug doses in mental health nursing

People with mental-health-related conditions should always be treated in the same way as others in your care and are often known as service users to avoid any of the unjustified stigma historically attached to conditions such as manic depression, bipolar disorder or Tourette's syndrome. As with patients in clinical or surgical wards, their conditions can be managed or alleviated with correct medication.

The following activity allows the opportunity to experience calculations carried out with the types of medication used in the treatment of people with mental health disorders.

Activity 5.6

1. Your patient Godfrey has been ordered olanzapine, an anti-psychotic used for his schizophrenia and bipolar 1 mania. His medication is to be given by intramuscular injection (IMI) due to his current mixed episodes associated with bipolar disorder. The consultant has ordered a dose of 6.5mg from your available stock of 2.5mg/ml. What volume should you draw?
2. Maria has schizophrenia and also endures the effects of Tourette's syndrome. She has been prescribed haloperidol in order to control her condition at a rate of 7.5mg per dose given three times a day. Her medication is available in stock ampoules of 5mg per 2ml. Given that she will need this medication for her entire respite stay of three days, calculate how much is required per dose and for the duration of her visit.
3. Bart has a major depressive disorder and he has been ordered selegiline transdermal treatment. The effective dosage range is between 6 and 12mg per 24 hours. Bart's doctor has recommended a dosage of 56mg, given over a period of a week in equal amounts. Calculate the volume of treatment to be given to Bart daily.

(Continued)

(Continued)

4. Madge has been ordered donepezil hydrochloride to assist in the treatment of her Alzheimer's disease. She will begin on a dose of 5mg per day for three weeks then 10mg for a further three weeks before starting on the maximum dosage of 23mg per day. What amount of donepezil hydrochloride will Madge have had in grams after an initial 12 weeks of treatment?

Chapter summary

Accurate drug calculation is an essential skill that nurses have to acquire during their training, before they can be entered on the professional register for nurses. This chapter has covered the basis for drug calculations for tablets and for drugs in liquid form to be taken orally or by injection. Doses of insulin and doses by body weight have been introduced; children's drug calculations by body weight will be covered later in Chapter 7.

Always check the prescription drawn up for a patient. If a dose is written in micrograms and the stock supplied is in milligrams you will need to convert milligrams to micrograms in order to calculate the dose required. It is usual to convert to the lowest level of unit. For all drug calculations, make sure that you have both stock strength and stock required in the same unit of measurement.

The next chapter will look at IV drip rates as some drugs are administered via an IV drip.

Useful websites

The following websites offer revision material that you can use to enhance your numeracy skills. If you need to revise any of the skills covered earlier, for example in Chapters 2 and 3, look at the web pages listed at the end of those chapters.

Tests and calculations

The following website is useful for drug calculations practice and is free for six months if you register. Try a free download first and register when you need to.

1. Drug calculations quiz page

    www.testandcalc.com/quiz/index.asp

Nursing Standard

The *Nursing Standard* has online guides and resources for subscribers.

2.   **https://rcni.com/nursing-standard**

Visit the online resources on your computer at **https://study.sagepub.com/ starkingskrause4e** or on your smart phone or tablet and gain access to:

- over 400 extra questions to check your learning and gain extra practice;
- links to useful websites that build on the skills introduced in this chapter;
- an interactive glossary of key terms.

Answers to the activities

Activity 5.1 (pages 79–80)

For questions 1–3, tablets in the medicine cabinet are of strength 5mg per tablet and the tablets are scored.

1.   The strength required is 2500mcg = 2.5mg and the stock strength is 5mg.

$$\frac{\text{Strength required}}{\text{Stock strength}} \times \text{One tablet}$$

$$\frac{2.5}{5} \times 1 \text{ tablet} = \frac{1}{2} \text{ tablet}$$

Or using the NHS mnemonic where you Need 2.5mg and you Have 5mg and the Stock is one tablet:

$$\frac{N}{H} \times \frac{S}{1} = \text{The correct dose for the patient}$$

$$\frac{2.5}{5} \times \frac{1 \text{ tablet}}{1} = \frac{1}{2} \text{ tablet}$$

So Jim Bow needs to take $\frac{1}{2}$ tablet to get 2500mcg of warfarin as required.

Alternatively you could convert both to micrograms to remove the decimal point:

2.5mg = 2500mcg and 5mg = 5000mcg so the formula is = $\frac{2500}{5000} \times \frac{1 \text{ tablet}}{1} = \frac{1}{2}$ tablet.

2.   The strength required here is 7.5mg and the stock strength is 5mg so Jess Rarebit needs

$$\frac{7.5}{5} \times \frac{1 \text{ tablet}}{1} = 1\frac{1}{2} \text{ tablets.}$$

3. Since the stock strength is 5mg and the stock required is 0.005g we need to convert both to milligram before using the formula. See Chapter 3 on how to do conversions if you need some revision here.

$$0.005g = 5mg \text{ so the formula is } \frac{5}{5} \times \frac{1 \text{ tablet}}{1} = 1 \text{ so Alf Ensafety needs 1 tablet.}$$

For questions 4–6, tablets in the medicine cabinet are of strength 2mg per tablet and the tablets are scored.

4. The strength required here is 0.005g = 5mg and the stock strength is 2mg, the formula is

$$\frac{5}{2} \times \frac{1 \text{ tablet}}{1} = 2.5 \text{ so Pur Feck needs } 2\frac{1}{2} \text{ tablets.}$$

5. The strength required here is 2000mcg and the stock strength is 2mg, so the formula is

$$\frac{2}{2} \times \frac{1 \text{ tablet}}{1} = 1 \text{ so Fan Tessie needs 1 tablet.}$$

6. The strength required here is 5mg and the stock strength is 2mg and the formula is

$$\frac{5}{2} \times \frac{1 \text{ tablet}}{1} = 2\frac{1}{2} \text{ so Fatma Dyet needs } 2\frac{1}{2} \text{ tablets.}$$

For questions 7–9, tablets in the medicine cabinet are of strength 50mg per tablet and the tablets are scored.

7. The strength required here is 0.075g and the stock strength is 50mg so we need to convert to mg before using the formula. See Chapter 3 on how to do conversions if you need some revision here.

$$0.075g = 75mg \text{ so the formula is } \frac{75}{50} \times \frac{1 \text{ tablet}}{1} = 1.5 \text{ so James Glu needs } 1\frac{1}{2} \text{ tablets.}$$

8. The strength required here is 25mg and the stock strength is 50mg. $\frac{25}{50} \times \frac{1 \text{ tablet}}{1} = 0.5$ so Uri Kiddin needs $\frac{1}{2}$ tablet.

9. The strength required here is 0.15g and the stock strength is 50mg so we need to convert to mg before using the formula. See Chapter 3 on how to do conversions if you need some revision here. $0.15g = 150mg$ so the formula is $\frac{150}{50} \times \frac{1 \text{ tablet}}{1} = 3$ so Noah Way needs 3 tablets.

If you got the arithmetic incorrect here you may wish to refer back to Chapter 2 on using fractions, or to Chapter 3 on conversions. You could also look at the web pages listed at the end of those chapters for further practice. Remember that you are multiplying, not adding, here; this is a common error that can harm patients, so be careful.

Activity 5.2 (pages 82–3)

1. The stock required and the stock strength are in different units so we first convert them to the same units. 1.5g = 1500mg (see Table 5.1 for conversions). The 250mg/ml means that there is 250mg per millilitre of mixture.

$$\frac{1500}{250} \times \frac{1}{1} \quad \text{so Jill needs 6ml for her dose.}$$

2. $$\frac{750}{500} \times \frac{2}{1} \quad \text{so Patrick needs 3ml per dose.}$$

He has four doses per day so his total dosage is $4 \times 3 = 12$ml.

3. $\dfrac{600}{150} \times \dfrac{2.5}{1}$ so Amelia needs 10ml per dose.

4. $\dfrac{625}{125} \times \dfrac{1.5}{1}$ so Tawdry needs 7.5ml per dose.

   She has three doses per day so her total dosage is $3 \times 7.5 = 22.5$ml.

Activity 5.3 (page 86)

For questions 1–3, morphine is of 15mg/ml in the medicine cabinet.

1. The strength required (Need) is 0.15g. Notice here that the amount prescribed and the stock on hand are in different units so we need to convert both to milligrams, using Table 5.1.

   $0.15g = 150$mg

   So the stock strength (Have) is 15mg, the volume of stock solution (Stock) is 1ml.

   $\dfrac{150}{15} \times \dfrac{1}{1} = 10$ml

   So you need to select the 10ml syringe to draw up the 10ml required for Harpa's injection.

2. The strength required is 6mg, the stock strength is 15mg and stock volume is 1ml.

   $\dfrac{6}{15} \times \dfrac{1}{1} = 0.4$ml

   Select the 1ml syringe and draw up 0.4ml of morphine for Happie.

3. The strength required is 22.5mg, the stock strength is 15mg and stock volume is 1ml.

   $\dfrac{22.5}{15} \times \dfrac{1}{1} = 1.5$ml

   So select the 2ml syringe and draw up 1.5ml of morphine for Whats.

For questions 4–6, pethidine is of 100mg/2ml in the medicine cabinet.

4. The strength required is 0.3g, the stock strength is 100mg and stock volume is 2ml. In this case the units are different so you need to convert them both to milligrams, using Table 5.1.

   $\dfrac{300}{100} \times \dfrac{2}{1} = 6$ml

   So select the 10ml syringe and draw up 6ml of pethidine for Janice.

5. The strength required is 65mg, the stock strength is 100mg and stock volume is 2ml.

   $\dfrac{65}{100} \times \dfrac{2}{1} = 1.3$ml

   So select the 2ml syringe and draw up 1.3ml of pethidine for Pep.

6. The strength required is 87mg, the stock strength is 100mg and stock volume is 2ml.

   $\dfrac{87}{100} \times \dfrac{2}{1} = 1.74$ml

   So we select the 2ml syringe and draw up 1.74ml of pethidine for Crystal.

For questions 7–9, cortisone is of 125mg/5ml in the medicine cabinet.

7. The strength required is 0.06g, the stock strength is 125mg and stock volume is 5ml. In this case the units are different so you need to convert them both to milligrams, using Table 5.1.

$$\frac{60}{125} \times \frac{5}{1} = 2.4\text{ml}$$

So select the 3ml syringe and draw up 2.4ml of cortisone for Bren.

8. The strength required is 150mg, the stock strength is 125mg and stock volume is 5ml.

$$\frac{150}{125} \times \frac{5}{1} = 6\text{ml}$$

So select the 10ml syringe and draw up 6ml of cortisone for Hugh.

9. The strength required is 75mg, the stock strength is 125mg and stock volume is 5ml.

$$\frac{75}{125} \times \frac{5}{1} = 3\text{ml}$$

So select either the 3ml or 5ml syringe and draw up 3ml of cortisone for Kiera.

Activity 5.4 (page 87)

1. Pauline Booker has been prescribed 60 units. The U.20 contains 20 units per ml strength, so you need that amount drawn up in the syringe.

    1ml = 20 units

    So draw up 3ml of U.20 into the syringe for injection.

    Maj Ick has been prescribed 30 units. The U.40 contains 40 units per ml.

    1ml = 40 units

    $\frac{1}{2}$ ml = 20 units

    So 30 units = $\frac{3}{4}$ ml = 0.75ml

    So you draw up 0.75ml of the U.40 insulin into the syringe for injection.

    An alternative way of calculating this is: 40 units = 1ml

    1 unit = $\dfrac{1}{40}$

    30 units = $\dfrac{1}{40} \times 30 = \dfrac{3}{4}$ ml

    This method will work for all insulin calculations.

2. The syringe is graduated for 40 units. The insulin that is available is U.20.

    To give 32 units of U.40 you need to double the dose.

    32 × 2 = 64 units

Activity 5.5 (pages 88–9)

1. Ben weighs 55kg and is prescribed 20mg per kg in body weight to be given in four equal doses. His total prescribed is 55 × 20 = 1100mg. For each dose you divide the total by 4 (i.e. number of doses per day) so 1100 ÷ 4 = 275mg = 0.275g.

2. Jens weighs 64kg and is prescribed 100mg per kg in body weight per day. Jen's total dosage is $64 \times 100 = 6400$mg per day. This is to be divided into doses to be given every 6 hours for the next 24 hours. The number of doses will be $24 \div 6 = 4$ doses per 24-hour period. $6400 \div 4 = 1600$mg so each dose is of 1600mg. So Jens has four doses at 6-hour intervals of 1600mg = 1.6g per dose.

    A common mistake made here is to divide the total dose of 6400mg by 6, the interval time between doses, rather than by 4, the number of actual doses. This would give $6400 \div 6 = 1066.667$mg, meaning the patient is given a greatly reduced dosage.

3. Okao weighs 72kg and is prescribed 50mg per kg in body weight per day. Total dosage per day is $72 \times 50 = 3600$mg. This is to be divided into four doses. So each dose is $3600 \div 4 = 900$mg = 0.9g.

Activity 5.6 (pages 89–90)

Much of the care you give as a mental health nurse may be given in the service user's environment, such as their home or assisted living accommodation. The location should have no bearing on the crucial requirement for total accuracy in your calculations, so although the location is different, the methods used to find the accurate dosage remain the same.

$$\frac{\text{Strength required}}{\text{Stock strength}} \times \text{Volume of stock solution}$$

Or using the NHS mnemonic:

$$\frac{N}{H} \times \frac{S}{1} = \text{The correct dose for the patient}$$

1. Using the formula we have

    $$\frac{6.5}{2.5} \times \frac{1}{1} = 2.6 \quad \text{So Godfrey needs 2.6ml per dose.}$$

2. Using the formula we have

    $$\frac{7.5}{5} \times \frac{2}{1} = 3$$

    So Maria needs 3ml per dose, given three times daily, which means she requires $3 \times 3 = 9$ml. Since Maria will be staying for three days you will need to have 9ml $\times 3 = 27$ml available during her stay.

    Total minimum medication required for three days is 27ml.

3. This question gave an amount to be taken by Bart over the week or seven days and asks for the daily dosage. You must simply divide the user's prescribed requirement by the length of time for which it has been ordered.

    $56 \div 7 = 8$mg/day is needed by Bart.

4. Madge suffers from Alzheimer's and her consultant needs to monitor her total consumption of the drug to ensure guidelines on the maximum dosage are maintained. Your task is to calculate the amount of drug taken in total for 12 weeks, but remember to convert your result to grams before reporting your finding.

    $(5 \times 7 \times 3) + (10 \times 7 \times 3) + (23 \times 7 \times 6) = 1281$mg = 1.281g

    Did you remember the dosage ordered was the daily amounts for each week?

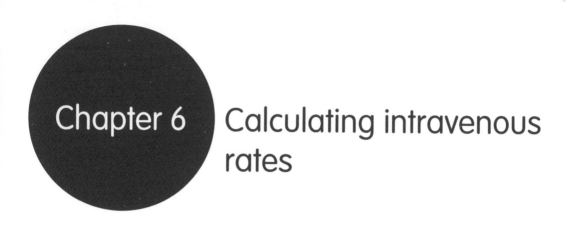

Chapter 6   Calculating intravenous rates

Chapter aims

By the end of this chapter you should be able to:

- calculate the flow rate in drops per minute that an intravenous infusion chamber should be set to in order to ensure an accurate delivery flow to individual patients;
- calculate the amount of time required for a volumetric infusion pump to deliver a given volume;
- calculate the flow rate required for a volumetric infusion pump to deliver a volume of fluid in a specified amount of time.

Introduction

These chapter aims may sound a little daunting, but you will soon become familiar with the terms used and understand the procedures. As a nurse you will need to be able to calculate the rate at which a fluid or medication is to be given to a patient by way of an intravenous (IV) infusion. It is a very common form of therapy, as you will see.

Case study

This extract is taken from the *Indian Journal of Pharmacology* (2010) and shows the importance of correct medication and observation.

A 7-month-old girl was referred with a history of high-grade fever for four days, lethargy, poor feeding for two days, hematochezia and ooze from IV puncture sites. The child was drowsy on examination with poor hemodynamic status, hepatomegaly, and free fluid in the abdomen. During illness she had received 5 doses of 250mg tablets of paracetamol, that is, 178 mg/kg/day (weight 7kg) along with 3 doses of 100mg of mefenamic acid per day (i.e. 43mg/kg/day). She was admitted in the ICU (intensive care unit) and given supportive therapy. She was given an IV loading dose of NAC. However, within 24 hours, her general condition deteriorated and she succumbed to multiorgan failure.

Some patients need a drug continuously, rather than in separate doses. One way of delivering medicine that way is by IV infusion; this is by infusing the drug in a liquid directly into a vein. As a student nurse, you will learn how to set up and calculate IV infusion rates.

IV infusion may also be used when a patient is unconscious and so cannot swallow. Some drugs and certainly blood transfusions always need to be delivered directly into the circulatory system. The registered nurse needs to be able to calculate the flow rate and the amount of time for the volume of drug/blood to be given.

Some patients that you see will require IV drugs that are keeping them alive. So errors that might not matter with some patients could be very serious for others. Most errors arise when the nurse makes mistakes in their calculations. It is like driving a car and breaking the speed limit; sometimes there is no adverse outcome, but on some occasions things go wrong and a tragedy occurs. What we can conclude from the report findings is that nurses need to make sure that all drugs administered via an IV are calculated correctly – and this chapter will show you how.

It is not only drugs that you, as a nurse, will assist in administering intravenously. It is very common in hospital to 'give fluids' this way. The fluids could be plasma or blood products needed after a patient loses blood during surgery or trauma such as a road traffic accident. Your patient may require replacement of body fluids lost for a variety of medical reasons, such as in cases of severe burns. Some patients will require an IV because they need to be hydrated, to prevent or lessen potential liver damage following an overdose of acetaminophen, or during a course of chemotherapy. The following case study is one where fluids given to a child had terrible consequences.

Case study

This story is taken from a South African newspaper and was published in November 2009 (*The Star*, 2009). Celina Kometsi took her 2-year-old daughter to her local hospital to be treated for burns on her hands. Two IV drips were inserted into the child's feet containing fluid which was infused for 3 hours. The child was reported to be in a great deal of pain and her feet started to swell and also turned purple.

A child's condition should always be monitored by a nurse and any problems, especially like the one above, should be reported to the doctor or consultant treating the patient. This story did not have a happy ending as the child had to have both her legs amputated just below the knee. Most IVs that you will be responsible for will not result in this serious condition but it does highlight the need for close monitoring.

In this chapter we will explain how to calculate the IV rate for two types of IV apparatus that are commonly used to give a patient their medication.

- In the first section we explain the calculation required to determine the rate of an IV using a **giving set** with **drip chamber**.
- In the second section you will learn to calculate the rate required using an IV **volumetric pump**.

When using the IV volumetric pump, you will need to be able to calculate the time required to deliver a volume of fluid, given the pump rate in millilitre per hour (ml/h). Activities on delivery rate required given the time to be taken will also feature in this chapter.

When you are tested on these calculations, you may not be allowed to use a calculator, so as you practise them you should attempt them without the aid of a calculator. Current recommendations from the Royal College of Nursing suggest that nursing students do not use calculators in their studies.

In Chapter 3 (Quantity conversions for nurses), you practised how to convert litres to millilitres. If you feel you need to revise this, go back to Chapter 3 and practise. You will need to understand that calculation for the activities in this chapter. IV calculations with a drip chamber set are done with the IV fluid amount in millilitre and so require conversion before calculation.

You may also want to review Chapter 2 (Essential numeracy requirements for nursing), as both cancelling down and the rounding of fractional or decimal values will also be used in this chapter.

Drip chamber giving sets

There are three main types of drip chamber or giving set in use throughout the healthcare system.

- **Macrodrip**: in which the chamber converts each millilitre of fluid into 15 drops; this is generally used for infusion of blood or other blood products such as **platelets** or **plasma**.
- Macrodrip: in which the chamber converts each millilitre of fluid into 20 drops; this is generally used for infusions such as normal saline or 5% dextrose.

The size of the drops is controlled by the fixed diameter of the plastic delivery tube. The drip rate delivered by each particular set is marked on the packaging of the IV giving set, so make sure that you select and use the correct drip size.

- **Microdrip**: in which the chamber converts each millilitre of fluid into 60 drops; this is generally used in critical care situations.

The giving set is the device used to break down the flow of each millilitre of fluid into droplets which can then be counted to ensure the correct number of droplets per minute for each of your patients. You should always ensure that you correctly identify the giving set to be used by *personally checking* its packaging. To correctly calculate the flow rate of the giving set with a drip chamber, follow this simple formula.

$$\text{IV flow rate} = \frac{\text{IV amount in ml} \times \text{giving set}}{\text{Hours} \times 60}$$

Notice that the bottom of the fraction is the time over which the IV is to be given in hours multiplied by 60. This is equivalent to the time in minutes. If the time over which the IV is to be given is already in minutes, you do not need to convert it to hours or multiply it by 60. If the time is given as hours and minutes, convert it to a total number of minutes; you do not need to multiply the result by 60. If you need practice with time conversions, revise Chapter 2.

Scenario

Nicola Burke has had surgery and is now regaining consciousness from the anaesthetic in the recovery ward. As you are on placement in Gerbera Ward you have been tasked to set up an IV for Nicola. The consultant has ordered 1 litre of Lactated Ringer's Solution over 8 hours using a 20 drops/ml Macrodrip set.

As the amount to be given is in litres, you will first need to convert this to millilitres. Chapter 3 (Quantity conversions for nurses) covers this in detail; revise this calculation if necessary. Having converted the IV amount to millilitres, put all the information into the formula.

$$\text{IV rate} = \frac{1000 \times 20}{8 \times 60}$$

This calculation can be cancelled down as shown in Chapter 2 (Essential numeracy requirements for nursing).

$$\text{IV rate} = \frac{125 \times 1}{1 \times 3} = \frac{125}{3} = 41\frac{2}{3} \text{ or } 41.66 \text{ drops/min}$$

As quite often occurs when calculating an IV rate, the numbers do not cancel out to an exact number of drops per minute. No matter how you try it is not usually possible to divide a droplet into a fraction or decimal, hence fractional and decimal answers require rounding. If you need to revise this skill, again refer back to Chapter 2.

The fraction $\frac{2}{3}$ or the decimal 0.66 is more than half way to the next whole number and so the answer is rounded up to 42.

The IV for Nicola needs to be set at 42 drops/minute to ensure she receives her prescribed IV over the period of time set.

You should try this chapter's activities without the aid of a calculator.

Activity 6.1

It has been a busy day in the operating theatre and the following patients have all arrived in the Gerbera Ward recovery room. Calculate the rate of the IV for each of the following patients for the amounts of Lactated Ringer's Solution listed. Each IV solution will be using a Macrodrip 20 drops/ml drip chamber giving set.

1. Charlie Cat 900ml over 5 hours
2. Mark Pain 1 litre over 6 hours
3. Olive Short 1.5 litres over 9 hours
4. Paris Walker 750ml over 4 hours
5. Amber Barton 500ml over 2 hours

Calculate the rate of the IV for each of the following patients for the amounts of Hartmann's Solution (CSL) listed. Each IV will be using a Macrodrip 20 drops/ml drip chamber giving set.

6. Mina Patel $\frac{1}{2}$ litre over 4 hours
7. Sharon Kite 750ml over $3\frac{1}{2}$ hours
8. Frank Smith $\frac{3}{4}$ litre over 6 hours 30 minutes
9. Noah Tablet $1\frac{1}{2}$ litres over 18 hours
10. Adam Stone 500ml over 2 hours 45 minutes

Answers to all the activities can be found at the end of the chapter.

For the infusion of blood, platelets or plasma, a Macrodrip chamber that converts each millilitre of fluid to be given into 15 drops/ml is most commonly used.

Scenario

Nazeem Ali has had a traffic accident and requires a blood plasma infusion. You are on placement in the Accident and Emergency Ward and have been tasked to set up the infusion for Nazeem. The **registrar** has ordered 750ml of plasma over 2 hours using a 15 drop/ml Macrodrip set.

As the amount to be given is in millilitres there is no need to convert before calculating the flow rate. Place the given information directly into the formula.

$$\text{IV flow rate} = \frac{750 \times 15}{2 \times 60}$$

This calculation can be cancelled down as shown in Chapter 2 (Essential numeracy requirements for nursing).

$$\text{IV rate} = \frac{375 \times 1}{1 \times 4} = \frac{375}{4} = 93\frac{3}{4} \text{ or } 93.75 \text{ drops/min}$$

Again, the IV rate does not cancel to an exactly even answer. The fraction $\frac{3}{4}$ or the decimal 0.75 is over half way to the next whole number and so the answer is rounded up to 94. Refer back to Chapter 2 for rounding fractions and decimals if needed.

The infusion for Nazeem needs to be set at 94 drops/min to ensure she receives her prescribed IV over 2 hours.

Activity 6.2

You are working on Sunshine Ward which cares for patients suffering with haemophilia at a day surgery. The patients today are to each receive a plasma product as part of their treatment. Calculate the IV rate for each of the following patients given their amounts of medication listed. Each IV will be delivered using a Macrodrip 15 drops/ml drip chamber giving set.

1. Julie Swan 500ml over 5 hours
2. Hussein Patel 1 litre over 6 hours
3. John Star $\frac{1}{2}$ litre over 4 hours
4. Lenny Short 400ml over 3 hours
5. Sarah Long $\frac{3}{4}$ litre over 7 hours

The third type of drip chamber is the Microdrip, which converts each millilitre of fluid into 60 drops. This chamber is commonly found in critical care settings.

Scenario

Heather has been rushed to hospital suffering from an accidental overdose of acetaminophen, a common ingredient of over-the-counter painkillers. After several hours in the Accident and Emergency (A&E) Department, Heather has been transferred to the critical care ward. You are required to install a new IV for Heather which delivers 1 litre of acetylcysteine over 16 hours using a Microdrip giving set drip chamber.

As the amount to be given is in litres you will first need to convert this amount to millilitres. Refer to Chapter 3 (Quantity conversions for nurses) for conversion of litres to millilitres if necessary. Having converted the amount to millilitres, put the information directly into the formula.

$$\text{IV flow rate} = \frac{1000 \times 60}{16 \times 60}$$

This calculation can be cancelled down as shown in Chapter 2 (Essential numeracy requirements for nursing).

$$\text{IV rate} = \frac{125 \times 1}{2 \times 1} = \frac{125}{2} = 62\frac{1}{2} \text{ or } 62.5 \text{ drops/min}$$

The fraction $\frac{1}{2}$ or the decimal 0.5 is half way to the next whole number and so is rounded up to 63. Refer back to Chapter 2 for rounding of fractions and decimals if necessary.

The IV for Heather needs to be set at 63 drops/minute to ensure she receives the IV amount prescribed over the correct time period.

Activity 6.3

Following a busy period in Woodlands Hospital A&E, the following patients have been transferred to the Carnation Critical Care Unit where you are on shift. Calculate the rate of IV infusion for each of the following patients using a Microdrip 60 drops/ml giving set drip chamber for the amounts of IV fluid shown.

1. Mercy Adebola 300ml over 3 hours
2. Glynis Sharp 500ml over 5 hours
3. Hilda James $\frac{1}{2}$ litre over 6 hours
4. Larry High 0.6 litre over 4 hours
5. Janet Snow 0.05 litre over 1 hour

Volumetric IV pump

The other most frequently used method of intravenous infusion is a volumetric pump. The pump is used to deliver rates of fluids at 5ml or more per hour in most nursing applications.

Scenario

Adeoti Khan is to receive 5% dextrose (D5W) over a period of ten hours following her collapse while running a marathon. The volumetric infusion pump has been set at a rate of 75ml/h. Calculate the amount of D5W she will receive during this period.

To calculate the amount of D5W received by Adeoti you need only to multiply the rate of infusion by the time the pump will be in use.

IV amount = Volumetric pump rate × Time in hours
IV amount = 75ml/h × 10 hours
$\qquad$ = 750ml

Activity 6.4

After a particularly hot day, several competitors from various sports have been brought to the surgery where you are working on placement. They are all suffering from dehydration and heat-related stress symptoms. The general practitioner has decided to put them all on rehydration IV treatment with D5W. Calculate the infusion amount in millilitres that each of the following competitors will receive.

1. Joline James $2\frac{1}{2}$ hours at 40ml/h
2. Paul Brook 3 hours at 60ml/h
3. Simon Payne 4 hours 15 minutes at 80ml/h
4. Graham Moore 1 hour 30 minutes at 50ml/h
5. Alan Gray 2 hours at 100ml/h

At times you may be required to calculate the time a volumetric pump will take to infuse a given amount of fluid at a predetermined or preset rate.

> ## Scenario
>
> ....
>
> Ari Shukla is receiving an infusion of 1.8 litres at the rate of 450ml/h. The consultant treating Ari would like to schedule some further tests for him and has asked you how long this infusion will take.

To calculate the amount of time Ari's IV will take you need to divide the amount to be infused by the rate of the volumetric pump. Since the rate per hour is in millilitres you will first need to convert the amount of the IV to millilitres, then divide this by the rate at which the volumetric pump is to be set.

$$\text{Time in hours for volumetric pump} = \frac{\text{IV in ml}}{\text{Pump rate}}$$

Refer to Chapter 3 (Quantity conversions for nurses) for conversion of litres to millilitres if necessary. Once the amount is converted to millilitres, put the figures directly into the formula. The calculation can then be cancelled as shown in Chapter 2 (Essential numeracy requirements for nursing), giving the number of hours the volumetric pump will require to infuse the prescribed amount of fluid.

$$\text{Length of time for IV} = \frac{1800}{450}$$
$$= 4 \text{ hours}$$

You can now inform the consultant that the pump will infuse the amount prescribed over 4 hours.

Activity 6.5

Your placement sees you working in a respite day centre for cancer patients. Some of the patients are due their chemotherapy treatments and these will be given today using a number of volumetric pumps. Calculate the time the patients will require to receive their IV amounts.

1. Stuart Mitchell 1 litre at 250ml/h
2. Sally Salone 1.5 litres at 200ml/h
3. Richard Goodey 1 litre at 300ml/h
4. Fay Fawcett 2.5 litres at 500ml/h
5. Abe Tamboya 0.75 litre at 200ml/h

There could be times when a patient is ordered an IV amount to be given by volumetric pump in a specific time. In such a scenario you would need to calculate the rate at which the pump should be set to ensure proper timely delivery of the IV amount. This situation might occur if a consultant has prescribed that a new mother is to receive an IV prior to her discharge from the maternity unit or birthing centre.

Scenario

Johanna Stewart is to receive an infusion of 1 litre Lactated Ringer's Solution over a period of 8 hours. You have the volumetric pump prepared and must now determine the rate to deliver the solution over the prescribed time period.

$$\text{IV volumetric pump flow rate} = \frac{\text{IV in ml}}{\text{Hours}}$$

The IV volume is in litres so convert the prescribed volume to millilitres. Refer to Chapter 3 (Quantity conversions for nurses) for conversion of litres to millilitres if necessary. Having converted the amount to millilitre, put the figures into the formula. The calculation will cancel down as shown in Chapter 2 (Essential numeracy requirements for nursing), giving the rate at which the volumetric pump should be set to ensure accurate timely delivery.

$$\text{IV volumetric pump rate} = \frac{1000}{8}$$

$$= 125\text{ml/hour}$$

Activity 6.6

As part of your training you are working in a birthing centre and caring for the new mothers following the birth of their children. As part of the recovery process, the Non-Medical Prescribing (NMP) Nurse in charge of the unit has ordered an IV of Lactated Ringer's Solution for the following new mothers. Calculate the rate at which each volumetric pump will be set to ensure the correct flow rate for delivery of the solution in the time prescribed.

1. Clare Rogers 1 litre over 2 hours
2. Martina Pye $\frac{1}{2}$ litre over 2 hours
3. Julie McIntyre $2\frac{1}{4}$ litres over 5 hours
4. Michaela Moore 2.25 litres over 6 hours
5. Simba Bengal 2 litres over 5 hours

Chapter summary

An essential skill that every nurse should acquire during their training is accuracy. This chapter has covered the calculation of rates of IV infusion to ensure that your patients receive their medication over the prescribed time period. The patient relies on receiving the correct amount of fluid at the correct rate for their recovery and treatment.

The skills you revised in Chapter 3 have been used to convert the required amount of fluid to be given into millilitres; your skills in cancelling down, multiplication, rounding and conversion of time fractions, practised in Chapter 2, have been used to ensure you reach the accurate flow rates.

Useful website

Test and calculations

The following website is useful for IV rate practice and is free for six months if you register. Try a free download first and register when you need to.

IV flow rates quiz

www.testandcalc.com/quiz/testiv.htm

References

Shivbalan, S, Sathiyasekeran, M and Thomas, K (2010) Therapeutic misadventure with paracetamol in children. *Indian Journal of Pharmacology*, 42: 412–15. Available online at: www.ijp-online.com/text.asp?2010/42/6/412/71894 (accessed 29 May 2012).

The Star, 28 November 2009. Available online at: www.iol.co.za/index.php?set_id= 1&click_id=125&art_id=vn20091128082542696C913737 (accessed 30 November 2009).

Visit the online resources on your computer at **https://study.sagepub.com/ starkingskrause4e** or on your smart phone or tablet and gain access to:

- over 400 extra questions to check your learning and gain extra practice;
- links to useful websites that build on the skills introduced in this chapter;
- an interactive glossary of key terms.

Answers to the activities

Activity 6.1 (page 100)

$$\text{IV rate} = \frac{\text{IV amount in ml} \times \text{giving set}}{\text{Hours} \times 60}$$

1. Charlie Cat 900ml over 5 hours

    $\dfrac{900 \times 20}{5 \times 60} = 60$ giving an IV rate of 60 drops/min

2. Mark Pain 1 litre over 6 hours

    $\dfrac{1000 \times 20}{6 \times 60} = 55.5$ giving an IV rate of 56 drops/min

3. Olive Short 1.5 litres over 9 hours

    $\dfrac{1500 \times 20}{9 \times 60} = 55.5$ giving an IV rate of 56 drops/min

4. Paris Walker 750ml over 4 hours

    $\dfrac{750 \times 20}{4 \times 60} = 62.5$ giving an IV rate of 63 drops/min

5. Amber Barton 500ml over 2 hours

    $\dfrac{500 \times 20}{2 \times 60} = 83.3$ giving an IV rate of 83 drops/min

6. Mina Patel $\frac{1}{2}$ litre over 4 hours

    $\dfrac{500 \times 20}{4 \times 60} = 41.6$ giving an IV rate of 42 drops/min

7. Sharon Kite 750ml over $3\frac{1}{2}$ hours

    $\dfrac{750 \times 20}{210} = 71.4$ giving an IV rate of 71 drops/min

8. Frank Smith $\frac{3}{4}$ litre over $6\frac{1}{2}$ hours

    $\dfrac{750 \times 20}{390} = 38.46$ giving an IV rate of 38 drops/min

9. Noah Tablet $1\frac{1}{2}$ litres over 18 hours

    $\dfrac{1500 \times 20}{18 \times 60} = 27.7$ giving an IV rate of 28 drops/min

10. Adam Stone 500ml over 2 hours 45 minutes

    $\dfrac{500 \times 20}{165} = 60.6$ giving an IV rate of 61 drops/min

Refer to Chapter 3 (Quantity conversion for nurses) for conversion of litres to millilitres if necessary. Refer to Chapter 2 for cancelling down as well as rounding of fractions and decimals if necessary.

Activity 6.2 (page 101)

$$\text{IV rate} = \frac{\text{IV amount in ml} \times \text{giving set}}{\text{Hours} \times 60}$$

1. Julie Swan 500ml over 5 hours

    $$\frac{500 \times 15}{5 \times 60} = 25 \text{ giving an IV rate of 25 drops/min}$$

2. Hussein Patel 1 litre over 6 hours

    $$\frac{1000 \times 15}{6 \times 60} = 41.6 \text{ giving an IV rate of 42 drops/min}$$

3. John Star $\frac{1}{2}$ litre over 4 hours

    $$\frac{500 \times 15}{4 \times 60} = 31.25 \text{ giving an IV rate of 31 drops/min}$$

4. Lenny Short 400ml over 3 hours

    $$\frac{400 \times 15}{3 \times 60} = 33.3 \text{ giving an IV rate of 33 drops/min}$$

5. Sarah Long $\frac{3}{4}$ litre over 7 hours

    $$\frac{750 \times 15}{7 \times 60} = 26.7 \text{ giving an IV rate of 27 drops/min}$$

If necessary, refer to Chapter 3 (Quantity conversions for nurses) for conversion of litres to millilitres, and to Chapter 2 for cancelling down and the rounding of fractions and decimals.

Activity 6.3 (page 102)

$$\text{IV flow rate} = \frac{\text{IV amount in ml} \times \text{giving set}}{\text{Hours} \times 60}$$

1. Mercy Adebola 300ml over 3 hours

    $$\frac{300 \times 60}{3 \times 60} = 100 \text{ giving an IV rate of 100 drops/min}$$

2. Glynis Sharp 500ml over 5 hours

    $$\frac{500 \times 60}{5 \times 60} = 100 \text{ giving an IV rate of 100 drops/min}$$

3. Hilda James $\frac{1}{2}$ litre over 6 hours

$$\frac{500 \times 60}{6 \times 60} = 83.3 \text{ giving an IV rate of 83 drops/min}$$

4   Larry High 0.6 litre over 4 hours

$$\frac{600 \times 60}{4 \times 60} = 150 \text{ giving an IV rate of 150 drops/min}$$

5. Janet Snow 0.05 litre over 1 hour

$$\frac{50 \times 60}{1 \times 60} = 50 \text{ giving an IV rate of 50 drops/min}$$

If necessary, refer to Chapter 3 (Quantity conversions for nurses) for conversion of litres to millilitres, and to Chapter 2 for cancelling down and the rounding of fractions and decimals.

Activity 6.4 (page 103)

IV amount = Volumetric pump rate × Time in hours

1. Joline James $2\frac{1}{2}$ hours at 40ml/h so 40 × 2.5 gives an infusion of 100ml
2. Paul Brook 3 hours at 60ml/h so 60 × 3 gives an infusion of 180ml
3. Simon Payne 4 hours 15 minutes at 80ml/h so 80 × 4.25 gives an infusion of 340ml
4. Graham Moore 1 hour 30 minutes at 50ml/h so 50 × 1.5 gives an infusion of 75ml
5. Alan Gray 2 hours at 100ml/h so 100 × 2 gives an infusion of 200ml

Refer to Chapter 2 for tips on multiplication.

Activity 6.5 (page 104)

$$\text{Time in hours for volumetric pump} = \frac{\text{IV in ml}}{\text{Pump rate}}$$

1. Stuart Mitchell 1 litre at 250ml/h so 1000 ÷ 250 will take 4 hours
2. Sally Salone 1.5 litres at 200ml/h so 1500 ÷ 200 will take $7\frac{1}{2}$ hours
3. Richard Goodey 1 litre at 300ml/h so 1000 ÷ 300 will take 3 hours 20 minutes
4. Fay Fawcett 2.5 litres at 500ml/h so 2500 ÷ 500 will take 5 hours
5. Abe Tamboya 0.75 litre at 200ml/h so 750 ÷ 200 will take 3 hours 45 minutes

If necessary, refer to Chapter 3 (Quantity conversions for nurses) for conversion of litres to millilitres, and to Chapter 2 for cancelling down and the conversion of time fractions or decimals.

Activity 6.6 (page 105)

$$\text{IV volumetric pump flow rate} = \frac{\text{IV in ml}}{\text{Hours}}$$

1. Clare Rogers 1 litre over 2 hours so $1000 \div 2$ will require a rate of 500ml/h

2. Martina Pye $\frac{1}{2}$ litre over 2 hours so $500 \div 2$ will require a rate of 250ml/h

3. Julie McIntyre $2\frac{1}{4}$ litres over 5 hours so $2250 \div 5$ will require a rate of 450ml/h

4. Michaela Moore 2.25 litres over 6 hours so $2250 \div 6$ will require a rate of 375ml/h

5. Simba Bengal 2 litres over 5 hours so $2000 \div 5$ will require a rate of 400ml/h

Refer to Chapter 2 for cancelling down if necessary.

Chapter 7 Calculations and children

Chapter aims

By the end of this chapter you should be able to:

- calculate the dose by weight of the child;
- calculate the dose required by the surface area of a child.

Introduction

You may well recognise that the Nursery and Midwifery Council (NMC) Standards and Essential Skills Clusters for children have already been seen in other chapters of this book. This should come as no surprise as children are in some respects smaller versions of your adult patients. One main difference comes in the range of sizes and weights of child patients compared to adults. If you are studying children's nursing then your patients could range in size from a premature baby as small as 500 grams through to an obese adolescent who may weigh as much as an adult.

The amount of medication an adult patient receives will offer no comparison to that given to a premature baby whose weight has been recorded at 0.52 kilograms. This weight could be as little as $\frac{1}{100}$ of the mother's weight. Complications during the birth could mean that both mother and child require treatment, but the potency of modern drugs and medicines means that the child's dose is not simply $\frac{1}{100}$ of the mother's prescription.

Case study

Magella has given birth to a daughter she has named Tuesday. The birth was complicated due to Magella having a serious lower respiratory tract infection. During the birth the registrar confirmed that Tuesday has contracted her mother's infection. Now

(Continued)

(Continued)

both Magella and Tuesday will require treatment for this infection. Magella has an allergy to penicillin and is to be treated with clindamycin. Since Tuesday is only a few days old and has not yet been tested for any allergic reaction she will be treated with the same drug for now. The drug being used is suitable for both adults and children.

As an adult, Magella will be treated at a prescribed dose of 450 milligrams given in two equal doses each day for five days. Tuesday is prescribed a paediatric dosage of 16mg/kg/day in four equal doses, due to her being a small premature baby weighing just 1.35 kilograms. The consultant **paediatrician** could have also prescribed Tuesday's medication using her body surface area of $0.06m^2$ and a prescription of $360mg/m^2$.

When prescribing medication for children, the dosages are often prescribed according to the patient's weight. This is due to the weight variance of child patients: from a premature baby who may weigh just 500 grams to an obese teenager weighing as much as 60 kilograms or more, child patients can vary greatly in size and weight. Some adult medications are also ordered using the patient's weight; the methods used to calculate these dosages are the same for both adults and children.

By the end of this chapter you should be able to accurately calculate the dosage requirement of any patient, no matter their age, given their weight. As in Chapter 5 (Drug calculations), some activities may require conversion prior to calculation of the dose. These conversions are covered in Chapter 3 (Quantity conversions for nurses) and apply no matter the age or size of your patient. You may wish to revise Chapter 3 as well as Chapter 2 (Essential numeracy requirements for nursing), as both contain essential best-practice skills used in calculating children's medication amounts.

Calculation of dosage by weight

The ability of a nurse to accurately calculate the dosage that a patient under their care is to receive is a fundamental core skill required by all nurses.

Scenario

Grace Stark is 5 years of age and suffers from focal epileptic seizures. Grace must take primidone tablets to keep her seizures under control. The tablets have been ordered as 20mg/kg/day to be taken in three equal doses. Grace weighs 18.75 kilograms. You must calculate the current correct daily dosage amount for this little girl and also how many tablets her mother is to give her for each single dose. Scored tablets of strength 50 milligrams are currently available from the pharmacy supplying Grace's medication.

In this scenario you will need to use the skills you have practised in the previous chapters. You will use multiplication and division (Chapter 3) and then calculate the number of tablets Grace's mother will give her daughter each time (Chapter 5).

To calculate Grace's current daily dosage you must multiply her weight by the amount of milligrams ordered per kilogram.

$18.75 \times 20 = 375mg$

This figure is the daily amount in milligrams that Grace must take to control her seizures. This total daily dosage will then be divided into the three equal single doses.

$$\frac{1\ \ 2\ \ 5}{3\overline{)3\ ^07\ ^15}}$$

So Grace will require 125 milligrams three times daily. You can now calculate the correct number of tablets.

Need = 125mg; Have = 50mg; Stock = 1 tablet

The correct dose for Grace $= \dfrac{N}{H} \times \dfrac{S}{1}$

$\dfrac{125}{50} \times \dfrac{1}{1} = 2\dfrac{1}{2}$ tablets

You can now confidently inform Grace's mother that the single dose to be taken three times daily will be $2\dfrac{1}{2}$ tablets .

Hint ... When writing the answer to a drug calculation always remember to include the unit of measure in the answer. This will enable your peers to know exactly the amount of medication and the method of delivery, liquid in millilitres or in tablet form or as capsules, that you have calculated the patient should have, given the individual's prescription.

You should now attempt the following activities without the aid of a calculator.

Activity 7.1

You are on placement with the Community Nurse and attending children who have developed community-acquired pneumonia. The Community Nurse has trained to Non-Medical Prescribing (NMP) status and so is qualified to prescribe medication for the children. All the children range in age from 2 to 10 years and are prescribed 8mg/kg/day of levofloxacin.

Given the weight of each child, how much levofloxacin should each of them be given for their condition?

1. Adnan Hussein weighs 14.25kg
2. Chiara Marden weighs 23.65kg
3. Kat Moreton weighs 15.75kg
4. Michael Abraham weighs 23.3kg
5. Andrew Sims weighs 14.65kg
6. Charlie Simpson weighs 17.35kg

Answers to all the activities can be found at the end of the chapter.

Activity 7.2

While you are still on placement with the Community Nurse there is an outbreak of chickenpox. It has been decided that the infected children will be treated with valacyclovir hydrochloride at the dosage of 20mg/kg/day. The medication will be administered by each child's parent or guardian three times daily for five days.

Given the weight of each child, how much valacyclovir hydrochloride should each of them be given as a daily dose for their chickenpox?

1. Simon Michelle weighs 7.5kg
2. Phil Crompton weighs 24.7kg
3. Mercy Grace weighs 18.33kg
4. Mohammed Murray weighs 16.46kg
5. Getcha Sumtime weighs 29.53kg

Activity 7.3

During your studies you have been allocated a placement on the Children's Ward at a major regional hospital. This particular ward specialises in renal patients. As part of their anaemia treatment the children on this ward are being treated with darbepoetin alpha. Each child will receive 2.25mcg/kg by **subcutaneous** injection weekly. Your task at the commencement of today's shift is to calculate the dosage to be drawn up for each child.

1. Harry Goldberg weighs 20.6kg
2. Gordonna Crunwell weighs 5.48kg
3. Toby Eddison weighs 12.4kg
4. Aces Orbetter weighs 9.56kg
5. Whatsup Hearannow weighs 24.16kg

There are some drugs, such as the cancer drug **dactinomycin**, which can be prescribed as either an amount per kilogram of patient weight or as an amount per square metre (m²) of body surface area (BSA) of the individual patient. In the next activity you are asked to calculate the amount of medication required using a patient's weight. The next section of this chapter covers BSA medication calculations; you will then calculate the drug dosage for the same patients using body surface area rather than weight.

Activity 7.4

The following children are being treated with dactinomycin for a **nephroblastoma**, a tumour of the kidneys that typically occurs in children. The **oncologist** treating the children has prescribed a medication cycle for each child at 15mcg/kg/day. As part of your daily duties you are asked to calculate each child's required dose.

1. Billy Bob weighs 20kg
2. Samantha Odeer weighs 16kg
3. Bethany Charleston weighs 28kg
4. Hyacinth Boukay weighs 26kg
5. Joaquin Johnes weighs 34kg

At the end of the next section these same five children will have their medication prescribed by their BSA.

Calculation of dosage by surface area

More commonly found in paediatric nursing is dosage by BSA. The BSA of a patient can be found using a commercially available chart known as a **nomogram**. These charts utilise a patient's height and weight to predict or estimate the surface area of the patient's body. Nomograms base the calculation of a patient's BSA on an assumption that the patient is of average weight for their height; obese patients could be measured using other methods. One alternative method of calculating a patient's BSA involves using the Mosteller formula. This formula was first published by the *New England Medical Journal* in 1987 and has been widely reprinted throughout the world in medical journals and texts. It is one of many published formulas that can be used to calculate the BSA of children or adults.

$$\text{BSA}(\text{m}^2) = \sqrt{\frac{\text{weight (kg)} \times \text{height (cm)}}{3600}}$$

The Mosteller formula, along with the other even more complex formulas that can be used to calculate a patient's BSA, will not be covered in this book.

The average BSA of children can vary from 0.25m² for **neonates** (newborn babies) up to 1.33m² for a preteen child. The averages for adults are 1.6m² for women and 1.9m² for men. With the ongoing development of new drugs to fight diseases, drug delivery methods could change in the future, potentially increasing the practice of prescription by BSA; the skills you practise here could be applied to any patient in your care.

Scenario

Adeana Begum has acute lymphoblastic leukaemia and is being treated with doxorubicin hydrochloride on a four-weekly cycle of intravenous infusion. Adeana has been prescribed a dose of 40mg/m² by her oncologist. With the use of the oncology ward's nomogram you have calculated Adeana's BSA at 1.15m².

You must now calculate the required amount of doxorubicin hydrochloride that she is to receive.

The calculation of dose by BSA is carried out in the same way as the calculation for dose by body weight. So again the skills gained in Chapter 2 (Essential numeracy requirements for nursing) of multiplying decimal numbers will be utilised. Should you feel it necessary, review Chapter 2 before attempting these Chapter 7 activities.

With the use of the nomogram you determined that Adeana has a surface area of 1.15m² and the oncologist ordered 40mg for every square metre. Therefore the calculation is 1.15 multiplied by 40.

$1.15 \times 40 = 46$

You now know that Adeana will require 46mg to be infused during this treatment session. Further treatment, if required, will be determined by her oncologist in 28 days.

Activity 7.5

During this placement you are working at a specialist children's hospital on the cancer ward. The children all attend a special hospital school while staying on the ward and so will be practising their multiplication skills with you. This encourages the children to keep up their studies while in hospital. As with all children, their age, heights and weights are all different and so you must calculate their individual dosages.

The oncologist for the ward is the same as Adeana's and has ordered 40mg of doxorubicin hydrochloride for every square metre of BSA for each child. Calculate the correct amount each of the children should receive given their BSA.

1. Penny Pharthing $0.75m^2$
2. Thomas Llandar $1.48m^2$
3. Iain Stuart $0.93m^2$
4. Ibrahim Mohamed $0.88m^2$
5. Itsa Oddity $1.54m^2$

Activity 7.6

Still working with the oncology department, you have moved across to another ward which treats the younger children. These children have been diagnosed with rhabdomyosarcoma, a childhood tumour that usually occurs only in children under 5. These children are being given vincristine sulfate injections dependent on their BSA as part of their treatment regime.

The paediatric oncologist has ordered each to be given $1.75mg/m^2$. You are tasked to undertake the calculations to determine each child's dose.

1. Katerina Whittle $0.72m^2$
2. Itz Mwa $0.48m^2$
3. Ima Troubell $0.60m^2$
4. Mohamed Mohamed $0.68m^2$
5. Geoff Dunnit $0.84m^2$

Activity 7.7

During your extended placement at the specialist children's hospital you have transferred to the paediatric heart ward. In this ward some of the children are suffering from **ventricular arrhythmias** that consultants have diagnosed as life threatening. As these children are all over the age of 2 they can be treated with sotalol which has been prescribed at 30mg/m² three times daily. You are asked by the Lead Nurse to calculate each child's dose given their individual BSA.

1. Richard Turiz 0.57m²
2. Copper Kettle 0.74m²
3. Keith Percival 0.83m²
4. Mader Nstink 0.92m²
5. Morris Woody 0.675m²

The children you met and nursed earlier on the oncology ward are now due their next round of medication. This time the children's doses are to be calculated using their BSA.

Activity 7.8

The following children are being treated with dactinomycin for a nephroblastoma. The oncology registrar treating the children has prescribed an intravenous five-day cycle of treatment for each child at 400mcg/m²/day. As part of your daily duties you are asked to calculate each child's required dose. This time their medication will be calculated using each child's BSA.

1. Billy Bob 0.75m²
2. Samantha Odeer 0.6m²
3. Bethany Charleston 1.05m²
4. Hyacinth Boukay 0.975m²
5. Joaquin Johnes 1.275m²

Chapter summary

Due to the size and often the fragility of your child patients, they are less likely to withstand any inaccuracy in their prescribed medications than adults. Accuracy is an essential, best-practice skill for every nurse, but it is particularly vital in the field of children's or paediatric medication because the values calculated are sometimes very small. Some of the patients you will treat will be too young to tell you where the pain is or that they require something such as a drink or to relieve themselves. These patients will need your best-practice skills and expertise at all times to aid their recovery from ailments or injuries. One day the child you nurse could be your nurse should you require nursing treatment in the future. Set them a good example of how the work of the nurse can improve life for everyone.

Visit the online resources on your computer at **https://study.sagepub.com/ starkingskrause4e** or on your smart phone or tablet and gain access to:

- over 400 extra questions to check your learning and gain extra practice;
- links to useful websites that build on the skills introduced in this chapter;
- an interactive glossary of key terms.

Answers to the activities

Activity 7.1 (page 114)

Given the weight of each child and the order for 8mg/kg/day, you need to multiply the weight by 8 to obtain the total daily dosage for each child.

1. Adnan Hussein requires $14.25 \times 8 = 114$mg
2. Chiara Marden requires $23.65 \times 8 = 189.2$mg
3. Kat Moreton requires $15.75 \times 8 = 126$mg
4. Michael Abraham requires $23.3 \times 8 = 186.4$mg
5. Andrew Sims requires $14.65 \times 8 = 117.2$mg
6. Charlie Simpson requires $17.35 \times 8 = 138.8$mg

Use the Hint. Whenever writing the answer to a drug calculation always remember to include the unit of measure for the answer. This will enable your peers to know exactly what amount of medication you have calculated that the patient should have.

Activity 7.2 (page 114)

The amount of valacyclovir hydrochloride each child should be given daily for their chickenpox is calculated by multiplying the given weight by the prescribed amount of 20 milligrams per kilogram.

1. Simon Michelle $7.5 \times 20 = 150$mg
2. Phil Crompton $24.7 \times 20 = 494$mg
3. Mercy Grace $18.33 \times 20 = 366.6$mg
4. Mohammed Murray $16.46 \times 20 = 329.2$mg
5. Getcha Sumtime $29.53 \times 20 = 590.6$mg

Remember the Hint and include the unit of measure in your answer to ensure everybody is clear about the exact dose for each patient. Should you feel you need to revise multiplying decimal numbers, refer to Chapter 2 (Essential numeracy requirements for nursing).

Activity 7.3 (pages 114–15)

Each child is to receive 2.25mcg/kg so to calculate the dosage for each child multiply their individual weight by 2.25.

1. Harry Goldberg requires $20.6 \times 2.25 = 46.35$mcg
2. Gordonna Crunwell requires $5.48 \times 2.25 = 12.33$mcg
3. Toby Eddison requires $12.4 \times 2.25 = 27.9$mcg
4. Aces Orbetter requires $9.56 \times 2.25 = 21.51$mcg
5. Whatsup Hearannow requires $24.16 \times 2.25 = 54.36$mcg

Remember the Hint and include the unit of measure in your answer to ensure everybody is clear about the exact dose for each patient. Should you feel you need to revise multiplying decimal numbers, refer back to Chapter 2 (Essential numeracy requirements for nursing).

Activity 7.4 (page 115)

For each child to receive 15mcg/kg/day you need to multiply their individual weights by 15.

1. Billy Bob requires $20 \times 15 = 300$mcg
2. Samantha Odeer requires $16 \times 15 = 240$mcg
3. Bethany Charleston requires $28 \times 15 = 420$mcg
4. Hyacinth Boukay requires $26 \times 15 = 390$mcg
5. Joaquin Johnes requires $34 \times 15 = 510$mcg

You may wish to revise Chapter 2 (Essential numeracy requirements for nursing) if you have any difficulties with multiplication. Remember the Hint and include the unit of measure in your answers to ensure everybody is clear about the exact dose for each patient.

Activity 7.5 (page 117)

The oncologist has ordered 40mg for every m² for each child, so multiply each child's surface area by 40.

1. Penny Pharthing requires $0.75 \times 40 = 30$mg
2. Thomas Llandar requires $1.48 \times 40 = 59.2$mg
3. Iain Stuart requires $0.93 \times 40 = 37.2$mg
4. Ibrahim Mohamed requires $0.88 \times 40 = 35.2$mg
5. Itsa Oddity requires $1.54 \times 40 = 61.6$mg

Remember the Hint and include the unit of measure in your answer to ensure everybody is clear about the exact dose for each patient. Should you feel you need to revise multiplying decimal numbers, refer to Chapter 2 (Essential numeracy requirements for nursing).

Activity 7.6 (page 117)

The paediatric oncologist ordered 1.75mg/m² so multiply each child's surface area by 1.75.

1. Katerina Whittle requires $0.72 \times 1.75 = 1.26$mg
2. Itz Mwa requires $0.48 \times 1.75 = 0.84$mg
3. Ima Troubell requires $0.60 \times 1.75 = 1.05$mg
4. Mohamed Mohamed requires $0.68 \times 1.75 = 1.19$mg
5. Geoff Dunnit requires $0.84 \times 1.75 = 1.47$mg

Revise the multiplication of decimal numbers in Chapter 2 (Essential numeracy requirements for nursing) if you feel it necessary. Remember to include the unit of measure in your answers so your peers are clear about the exact dose for each patient.

Activity 7.7 (page 118)

As the children are being treated with a prescription of 30mg/m², multiply each BSA by 30 to obtain the correct dose.

1. Richard Turiz requires $0.57 \times 30 = 17.1$mg
2. Copper Kettle requires $0.74 \times 30 = 22.2$mg
3. Keith Percival requires $0.83 \times 30 = 24.9$mg
4. Mader Nstink requires $0.92 \times 30 = 27.6$mg
5. Morris Woody requires $0.675 \times 30 = 20.25$mg

Remember the Hint and include the unit of measure in your answer to ensure everybody is clear about the exact dose for each patient. Should you feel you need to revise multiplying decimal numbers, refer back to Chapter 2 (Essential numeracy requirements for nursing).

Activity 7.8 (page 118)

Each child is to receive 400mcg/m²/day, so multiply their BSA by 400 to calculate each child's dose.

1. Billy Bob requires $0.75 \times 400 = 300$mcg
2. Samantha Odeer requires $0.6 \times 400 = 240$mcg
3. Bethany Charleston requires $1.05 \times 400 = 420$mcg
4. Hyacinth Boukay requires $0.975 \times 400 = 390$mcg
5. Joaquin Johnes requires $1.275 \times 400 = 510$mcg

The daily requirement of each child is the same as that when the dose was calculated using their weight. You may wish to revise the multiplication of decimal numbers using Chapter 2 (Essential numeracy requirements for nursing). Remember to include the unit of measure in your answers to ensure everybody is clear about the exact dose for each patient.

Chapter 8 Exam skills and revision exercises

Chapter aims

At the end of this book you should be able to:

- display the numeracy skills required as a nurse;
- carry out the drug calculations required to administer medicines safely via appropriate routes in Fields of Nursing including specific requirements for children and other groups;
- display the skills required to cancel down fractions as found in nursing calculations;
- multiply decimal numbers by another decimal value as found in nursing calculations;
- divide decimal numbers by another decimal value as found in nursing calculations;
- convert fractions to decimals as found in nursing calculations;
- convert decimals to fractions as found in nursing calculations;
- convert time fractions and decimals to minutes to carry out calculations for nursing;
- round decimal and fraction values as appropriate to nursing calculations;
- convert a given weight, be it of a drug or person, into a greater or lesser unit of weight measure in the metric system of measure as typically found in healthcare;
- convert a liquid measure from litres to millilitres and from millilitres to litres;
- convert a given length into a lesser or greater unit of length measure in the metric system of measurement as typically found in healthcare;
- multiply any amount by 10, 100, 1000;
- record fluid intake as required for healthcare calculations;
- record fluid output as required for healthcare calculations;
- complete a Fluid Balance Chart (FBC) for patient hydration care;
- provide a fluid balance value for a time period as required to evaluate a patient's hydration level;
- calculate the number of tablets required for patients from their prescription;
- calculate the dose required in liquid form as prescribed for a patient;

- calculate the drug dose prescribed for injection for a patient;
- calculate the drug dose for injection for patients requiring insulin;
- work out the dose to be given to a patient when prescribed by their body weight;
- calculate the flow rate in drops per minute that an intravenous (IV) infusion chamber should be set to ensure an accurate delivery flow to individual patients;
- calculate the amount of time required for a volumetric infusion pump to deliver a given volume of fluid to a patient;
- calculate the flow rate required for a volumetric infusion pump to deliver a volume of fluid in a specified amount of time.

Introduction

Revision is an important part of your learning process and hence an essential part of your training. Revision helps to consolidate what you have learnt and should give you a better understanding of the knowledge required of you. Nursing students must pass numeracy and mathematical calculations tests as part of their course to ensure they are competent in this essential skill. There will be other tests of your skills during your training and some subjects are covered in the other books in the Learning Matters series *Transforming Nursing Practice*. This chapter contains some helpful tips and advice to aid your revision gathered from both authors' years of experience as both students and teachers.

Revision techniques

Ideally the process of revision starts when you first meet the study materials in your class. The easiest way to learn, particularly for nursing calculations, is by doing plenty of examples and asking your tutor(s) questions about any problems as your studies progress. The purpose of revision is for you to check and to ascertain what you have understood and revise to consolidate your learning. For revision on any assessed work make sure you have the following.

- The up-to-date syllabus for your course that you are being assessed on. This is so you know what is required and identify all key areas that will be assessed.
- Your course notes with any examples given by your tutor. These can be used to help you, if you need to revise, when you get stuck on a particular topic. Be sure your notes are legible and if necessary rewrite them after the lectures to ensure you understand them. Try using separate folders for each subject to keep subject notes together.

- Any text or reference books you have used during the course, especially your copy of *Passing Calculations Tests in Nursing*. Having examples of the specialised requirements for your course that can be referred to when needed will be helpful.
- Specimen or past test papers, if available, for the specific course you are following. Always good to see what has been asked on previous test papers and make sure that examples you have are related to your course.
- Plenty of pens and paper for you to practise the revision questions and remember a bottle of water to keep you hydrated.
- Somewhere quiet to do your revision, either at home, university, public library or work place where you can study without being interrupted.
- A self-promised reward for yourself at the end of each revision session. It will help to motivate you as all students can get fed up at some stage and self-rewards or an indulgence can often help.

Getting started with revision can be difficult but try to schedule time to revise your coursework regularly. Revision involves you attempting any activity questions or coursework as set for your individual course or just redoing the activities found in this book. Identify the subjects or topics that you feel need revision, then seek help by looking back at your course notes or try re-reading the specific chapter in this book. When making your study timetable, remember to put in some revision slots and also some 'you' time to enjoy yourself as this often helps; not too much though. Half an hour spent revising questions or highlighting information by revisiting the chapters in this book or writing down a question you need to ask your tutor is better than two hours spent worrying about what to do and aimlessly reading, hoping some answer will suddenly arrive. You might also find it useful to revise with a friend, to talk problems through and test each other. If so, schedule some time when you both can work together.

The following case studies use the nursing best-practice skills that have been covered in this book. The case studies are based in hospital situations as the majority of nurses do the biggest proportion of their practical training in this environment. Read the following practice case studies and before attempting to answer the questions ask yourself the following.

- Do I understand what is being asked?
- Can I break down each case study into various tasks?
- Can I find all the relevant information here?
- Can I answer all or some of this, or should I revise the relevant chapter(s)?

If you answer yes to all of these, then attempt each case study in turn. Remember you can always revise a chapter or chapters in order to grasp the required mathematics. The answers to each case study can be found at the end of the chapter, and will refer you back to relevant chapters for further clarification and help.

For example, if you find you are unsure about filling out the Fluid Balance Chart, it is suggested that you revise Chapter 4 then re-attempt the particular case study.

Practice case study 8.1: A case study for a neonate patient

Lucy Mather is 20 weeks old and has been admitted to Buttercup Ward in the Woodland Hospital with respiratory and heart problems. She has been put on close monitoring of her fluid intake and output using a Fluid Balance Chart (FBC). All dry nappies for Lucy weigh 25g. Her NHS number is 132465 and her date of birth is 25 May 2017. Complete an FBC for her, using the practice FBC in Chapter 4's appendix (page 73).

Lucy's nappy was changed at the following times:

Time	Weight (g)
0600	165
0730	130
1200	145
1730	134
2100	184

Add the amount of urine passed to Lucy's FBC.

Lucy was given feeds of SMA milk:

Time	Amount (ml)
0500	120
0900	135
1315	120
1730	130
2130	100

Add these to Lucy's FBC.

a. Now work out Lucy's fluid balance.
b. At 1730 Lucy was fed, see above for the amount she took, and the bottle had 170ml at the start of her feed.

How much SMA did Lucy leave in the bottle?

c. On admission Lucy had a head circumference 44.1cm and weighed 6.53kg and during her stay at the Woodland Hospital she gained a further 120g.

(Continued)

(Continued)

What is her weight following this weight gain?

d.   At birth Lucy had a head circumference of 34cm and weighed 3.75kg.

How much weight had Lucy gained by the time she was admitted to Buttercup Ward? By how much had Lucy's head circumference increased?

e.   The consultant has asked you to record Lucy's heart rate at midday. You record 201 beats in 90 seconds.

What is Lucy's heart rate per minute?

f.   Her temperature at midday was 36.9° and at 6 p.m. is 37.5°.

How much has Lucy's temperature increased?

g.   Lucy is prescribed Lanoxin, to slow her heart beat, at 0.02mg/kg/every 6 hours. Lanoxin has stock strength of 0.5mg/2ml in the medicine cabinet. Calculate the volume for each dose.

Prepare the FBC and answers to the questions being asked for the consultant.

The next case study for you to practise takes elements of the mathematical calculations from the book and required as best practice by all healthcare professionals.

Practice case study 8.2: A case study for an adult patient

Susan Stay (date of birth 24 October 1952 and NHS number 73524) has just had major surgery for endometrial cancer and arrived on Foxglove Ward to regain consciousness from the anaesthetic. As you are on placement in the ward part of your duties today will be to set Susan's IV drip rate.

a.   The surgeon has prescribed 1 litre of Hartmann's Solution using a 20 drop/ml drip chamber giving set over 5 hours. Calculate the rate which should be set.

When Susan is moved to the surgical Hopewell Ward to continue her recovery you are transferred to the same ward. You will now carry out some of her care requirements over the course of your next shifts.

b.   Create a Fluid Balance Chart (FBC) for the hours between 8 a.m. and 3 p.m. given the following fluid measurements taken. Susan is also receiving an IV of 1 litre Lactated Ringer's Solution being given over a period of 16 hours. The IV is currently being infused using a 20 drop/ml drip chamber giving set and was commenced at 8 a.m. Be sure to include the IV drip she is receiving in your calculations.

0800	Tea	325ml		
0915			Urine	375ml
1000			Vomit	205ml
1100	Juice	200ml		
1230			Urine	220ml
1400	Water	150ml		
1400			Urine	265ml
1600	Water	200ml	Urine	135ml

c. Having completed the FBC, what is Susan's balance in millilitres?

d. What time is Susan's IV of Lactated Ringer's Solution due to be completed?

e. What is the correct rate for the drip chamber giving set to ensure this is achieved?

f. Susan is experiencing severe discomfort following her surgery and the registrar has prescribed apomorphine. The prescription states she should receive 4 milligrams of apomorphine. The drug is available on Hopewell Ward in strength of 0.04g/ml. You must now calculate the correct dose to be given to Susan.

g. As part of her medication Susan is to receive mitoxantrone injections every 21 days. The mitoxantrone has been prescribed at $12mg/m^2$ for Susan who has a body surface area (BSA) of $1.5m^2$. Calculate the amount of mitoxantrone she is to receive given the drug is available in strength 2mg/ml.

h. After discharge from hospital Susan was found to have deep vein thrombosis and is to be treated with Clexane injections given daily. The Clexane is to be given intramuscularly and is prescribed on body weight. Susan was weighed and this was recorded as 80 kilograms. The dosage prescribed is 1.5mg/kg/day. The drug is available in Pre-Filled Syringes of strength 20mg, 40mg, 60mg, 80mg and 100mg, and you are tasked to calculate how many injections and of what strength Susan should be given daily so that she receives the correct amount of Clexane each day.

Non-Medical Prescribing Nurse

During your career as a nurse you have cared for many patients and a possible logical progression in your career might be to become a Non-Medical Prescribing (NMP) Specialist. This is a relatively new position for nurses that have completed a post-graduate course and been licensed to issue medications to patients without a doctor present or needing to assess the patient. The qualification is issued to experienced nurses following a unit of post-graduate study, and in terms of drug calculation requires 100% accuracy in the final examination. During this time-limited test, generally no drug names are used so there is little possibility of nurses falling into a 'this drug so this much' answer and instead relies on making nurses think more.

The following exercises are some practice tests for this NMP course. When practising with these examples, be sure to observe a limit of 30 minutes per test. The aim is to help you, the experienced nurse, to better understand the pressure of an academic timed test. Remember, the more practice you have should help you to become faster and give you a better understanding of what is being asked. When you sit your finals, the result is all that matters and you will require a 100% result; anything less is a 'fail'.

Good luck and thank you for the care and dedication you have shown us, your patients, throughout your career! The answers to these tests can be found at the end of this chapter.

NMP Test 1

Maximum time 30 minutes. 100% pass rate only

Q1 Drug Z is available as 2.5 milligram tablets. The dose is 7.5 milligrams daily for one week followed by 10 milligrams daily for three weeks.

How many **tablets** would you prescribe for four weeks' supply?

Q2 Drug W is available as 750 milligrams/5 millilitres intravenous injection. A patient needs 1.5 grams of drug W per dose.

How many **millilitres** will you prescribe for each dose?

Q3 You need to prescribe Drug D to a child weighing 12.5 kilograms. Your patient needs 100mg/kilogram/day of Drug D in two divided doses.

How much Drug D will you have to prescribe per dose?

Q4 Drug L is available as 20 microgram tablets. The dose is 0.02 milligrams once a day. How many **tablets** would you need to prescribe for 28 days?

Q5 The dose of medicine for a child is 100 micrograms/kilogram body weight/day. Calculate the total daily dose needed in **milligrams** for a child weighing 23 kilograms.

NMP Test 2

Maximum time 30 minutes. 100% pass rate only

Q1 Drug M is available as 2.25 milligram tablets. The dose is 4.5 milligrams daily for one week followed by 6.75 milligrams daily for three weeks.

How many **tablets** would you prescribe for two weeks' supply?

Q2 Drug J is available as 625 milligrams/5 millilitres intravenous injection. A patient needs 1.5 grams of Drug J per dose.

How many **millilitres** will you prescribe for each dose?

Q3 You need to prescribe Drug E to a child weighing 12.5 kilograms. Your patient needs 100 mg/kilogram/day of Drug E in two divided doses.

How much Drug E will you have to prescribe per dose?

Q4 Drug K is available as 25 microgram tablets. The dose is 0.025 milligrams once a day. How many **tablets** would you need to prescribe for 21 days?

Q5 The dose of medicine for a child is 75 micrograms/kilogram body weight/day.

Calculate the total daily dose needed in **milligrams** for a child weighing 25 kilograms.

NMP Test 3

Maximum time 30 minutes. 100% pass rate only

Q1 Drug B is available as 3.5 milligram tablets. The dose is 7 milligrams daily for one week followed by 1.75 milligrams daily for three weeks.

How many whole **tablets** would you dispense for three weeks' supply?

Q2 Drug R is available as 375 milligrams/3 millilitres intravenous injection. A patient needs 1 gram of drug R per dose.

How many **millilitres** will you prescribe for each dose?

Q3 You need to prescribe Drug F to a child weighing 15.5 kilograms. Your patient needs 100mg/kilogram/day of Drug F in two divided doses.

How much Drug F will you have to prescribe per dose?

Q4 Drug K is available as 50 microgram tablets. The dose is 0.025 milligrams once a day.

How many **tablets** would you need to prescribe for 14 days?

Q5 The dose of medicine for a child is 50 micrograms/kilogram body weight/day.

Calculate the total daily dose needed in **milligrams** for a child weighing 25 kilograms.

NMP Test 4

Maximum time 30 minutes. 100% pass rate only

Q1   Drug B is available as 0.006 gram tablets. The dose is 6 milligrams daily for two weeks followed by 12 milligrams daily for 14 days.

How many **tablets** would you prescribe for **four** weeks' supply?

Q2   Drug R is available as 625 milligrams/2 millilitres intravenous injection. A patient needs 1 gram of drug R per dose.

How many **millilitres** will you prescribe for each dose?

Q3   You need to prescribe Drug F to a child weighing 27.5 kilograms. Your patient needs 100mg/kilogram/day of Drug F in two divided doses.

How much Drug F will you have to prescribe per dose?

Q4   Drug K is available as 50 microgram tablets. The dose is 0.075 milligrams once a day.

How many **tablets** would be needed for 21 days?

Q5   The dose of medicine for a child is 45 micrograms/kilogram body weight/day.

Calculate the total daily dose needed in **milligrams** for a child weighing 27 kilograms.

NMP Test 5

Maximum time 30 minutes. 100% pass rate only

Q1   Drug Z is available as 0.015 gram tablets. The dose is 30 milligrams daily for two weeks followed by 15 milligrams daily for 14 days.

How many **tablets** would you prescribe for the total **four** weeks' supply?

Q2   Drug W is available as 375 milligrams/3 millilitres intravenous injection. A patient needs 0.5 grams of drug W per dose.

How many **millilitres** will you prescribe for each dose?

Q3 You need to prescribe Drug D to a child weighing 34.4 kilograms. Your patient needs 10mcg/kilogram/day of Drug D in two divided doses.

How much Drug D will you have to prescribe per dose?

Q4 Drug D is available as 0.02 microgram tablets. The dose is 40 nanograms twice a day.

How many **tablets** would you need to prescribe for ten days?

Q5 The dose of medicine for a child is 40 micrograms/kilogram body weight/day.

Calculate the total daily dose needed in **milligrams** for a child weighing 13.25 kilograms.

More exercises like these will be available via the book's website; remember, the practice tests are designed to encourage thinking and problem solving before your finals.

Exam tips

The exam tips listed below give some advice on how to survive and do well in assessments tasks.

- Always check your learning timetable for any assessments. You need to know what time it is to be taken or submitted.
- If you are going to do a written assessment, always organise yourself regarding what you need to submit or take with you. For example, have your identity card, pens and pencils ready to hand.
- Arrive at least 10 minutes early at the assessment centre for any written test.
- Before undertaking any of your assessed tasks, have a good night's sleep, making sure you have a reliable alarm clock or someone to wake you up in plenty of time.
- Have something to eat and allow lots of time to travel, leaving early to arrive on time, to the examination centre/lecture hall where you will be assessed.
- Remember to listen to and/or read any instructions given to you by the invigilators and answer every question as fully as you can.
- Attempt all the questions required, taking careful note of the time you have allowed for each question. Do not spend too long on any one question.
- Move to another question if you get stuck on a particular question as you can always come back to this question if you have time before the end of the examination.
- Some examinations will give you a choice of questions, so make sure you read the instructions on the number of questions to answer – you may not have to do them all.

- See assessments as a chance to show off what you know; by now you have done plenty of revision and practice questions.

- Promise yourself a reward after the assessment so you have something to look forward to afterwards. I always found this was a good motivator for me!

Chapter summary

This chapter covers a variety of numerical tasks and mathematical tasks which nurses and other specialist nurses may be required to perform. By the time you reach this part of the book, you should have done some revision and you are ready to do your coursework-assessed tasks.

Good luck with your assessments and from all your prospective patients and service users, we thank you for caring for us.

Visit the online resources on your computer at **https://study.sagepub.com/ starkingskrause4e** or on your smart phone or tablet and gain access to:

- over 400 extra questions to check your learning and gain extra practice;
- links to useful websites that build on the skills introduced in this chapter;
- an interactive glossary of key terms.

Answers to the practice case studies

Practice case study 8.1 (pages 125–6)

The FBC in Figure 8.1 shows how you should have filled in the chart.

a. Fluid Balance Charts were covered in Chapter 4 so please look at this chapter for revision if you need to.

Lucy's dry nappy weighs is 25g so remember to take this off the total weight of her wet nappy to get the correct amount of urine passed. For example, for 0600 hours, the amount of urine is $165 - 25 = 140$ml.

Time	Weight (g)	Amount of urine (ml)
0600	165	140
0730	130	105
1200	145	120
1730	134	109
2100	184	159

Woodland Hospital	Clinical Skills Fluid Balance Chart	
Ward: *Buttercup*	Date: *12/10/17*	M/F: *F*
Family Name: *Mather*	First Name: *Lucy*	
NHS Number: *132465*	Date of Birth: *25/05/2017*	

| Time | INTAKE | | | | OUTPUT | | | | |
	By Mouth or Tube	ml	Intravenous	ml	Urine ml	Vomit or Tube	ml	Other	ml
0100									
0200									
0300									
0400									
0500	SMA	120							
0600					140				
0700					105				
0800									
0900	SMA	135							
1000									
1100									
1200					120				
1300	SMA	120							
1400									
1500									
1600									
1700	SMA	130			109				
1800									
1900									
2000									
2100	SMA	100			159				
2200									
2300									
2400									
Totals		605			633				
Total Input		605			Total Output		633		

Fluid Balance for time period = 605 − 633 = −28ml

Figure 8.1   Lucy Mather's FBC

Lucy's **Total output** is = 140 + 105 + 120+ 109 + 159 = 633ml and her **Total input** is 120 + 135 + 120 + 130 + 100 = 605ml.

Lucy's **Total fluid balance** = 605 − 633 = **−28ml**, that is she has a negative fluid balance so she passed more urine than she took in SMA milk.

Answer: Lucy's Total fluid balance = −28ml

b.   At 1730 Lucy was fed and she took 130ml of SMA milk. The bottle had 170ml at the start of her feed. There was 170 − 130 = 40ml of SMA milk left in the bottle.

Answer: 40ml of SMA milk left in the bottle

c.   On admission Lucy weighed 6.53kg and during her stay at the Woodland Hospital she gained a further 120g.

Note here that the two measurements are in different units so either use 120g = 0.120kg and add the two together, i.e. 6.53kg + 0.120kg = 6.65kg, or convert both units to grams and add together i.e. 6530g + 120g = 6650g and then convert back to kilograms to get 6.65kg.

Answer: Lucy's weight is now 6.65kg

Chapter 3 (Quantity conversion for nurses) can be used here to check how to convert kilograms to grams and vice versa if you need help on this.

d.   At birth Lucy weighted 3.75kg. She weighed 6.53kg on admission. To find how much weight she has gained we take her weight on admission and subtract her birth weight i.e. 6.53 − 3.75 = 2.78kg.

Answer: Lucy's weight gain by the time she was admitted to Buttercup Ward is 2.78kg

By how much had Lucy's head circumference increased?

At birth, Lucy had a head circumference of 34cm and on admission had a head circumference 44.1cm. To find out how much her circumference has increased we take her new circumference and subtract from it the birth circumference, i.e. 44.1 − 34 = 10.1cm.

Answer: Lucy's head circumference had increased by 10.1cm

e.   Lucy's heart rate at midday is 201 beats in 90 seconds. Now 90 seconds is one and a half minutes, so to get the rate per minute you divide 201 by 1.5 which is 134.

Answer: Lucy's heart rate per minute is 134

See Chapter 2 (Essential numeracy requirements for nursing) for help on division.

f.   Lucy's temperature at midday was 36.9° and at 6 p.m. it is 37.5°.

To find Lucy's temperature increase you subtract the midday reading from the 6 p.m. reading, i.e. 37.5 − 36.9 = 0.6°.

Answer: Lucy's temperature increased by 0.6°

g. Lucy is prescribed Lanoxin, to slow her heart beat, at 0.02mg/kg/every 6 hours. Lanoxin has stock strength of 0.5mg/2ml in the medicine cabinet. To get help with how to calculate the volume for each dose, see Chapter 5 on drug calculations.

Lucy's weight is now 6.65kg so she is to receive the following medication of Lanoxin:

$0.02 \times 6.65 = 0.133$mg every 6 hours.

For each dose we use the formula from Chapter 5. In this case

Need = 0.133mg = 133mcg   **H**ave = 0.5mg = 500mcg   **S**tock = 2ml

$$\frac{N}{H} \times \frac{S}{1} = \text{The correct dose for the patient}$$

$$\frac{133}{500} \times \frac{2}{1} = 0.532 \text{ ml}$$

Answer: Lucy needs 0.532ml per dose every 6 hours

Practice case study 8.2 (pages 126–7)

a. Susan is to receive an IV of 1 litre of Hartmann's Solution using a 20 drop/ml drip chamber giving set over 5 hours. You are to determine the drip rate at which the giving set should be set.

The calculation of IV rates is covered in Chapter 6 (Calculating intravenous rates), and you should refer back to this for revision.

$$\text{IV rate} = \frac{\text{IV amount in ml} \times \text{giving set}}{\text{Hours} \times 60}$$

$$\text{IV rate} = \frac{1000 \times 20}{5 \times 60} = 66.6$$

This figure must be rounded as seen in Chapter 2; as the decimal is over half way the amount will be rounded up.

Answer: IV rate 67 drops/minute

b. Remember Susan is receiving a litre of IV fluid over 16 hours. This requires you to calculate how much fluid is infused each hour, so refer to Chapter 2 (Essential numeracy requirements for nursing) for revision. Since 1 litre equals 1000 millilitres you will need to divide this by 16 to obtain the number of millilitres per hour. Refer to Chapter 2 for the division of numbers revision and to Chapter 3 (Quantity conversion for nurses) for revision on conversion of litre to millilitres.

$$\text{IV amount per hour} = \frac{1000}{16} = 62.5\text{ml}$$

This figure must appear each hour on your Fluid Balance Chart as it is part of Susan's fluid intake.

Woodland Hospital	Clinical Skills Fluid Balance Chart	
Ward: *Hopewell*	Date: *23/06/17*	M/F: *F*
Family Name: *Stay*	First Name: *Susan*	
NHS Number: *73524*	Date of Birth: *24/10/1952*	

Time	INTAKE By Mouth or Tube	ml	Intravenous	ml	Urine ml	OUTPUT Vomit or Tube	ml	Other	ml
0100									
0200									
0300									
0400									
0500									
0600									
0700									
0800	Tea	325	Ringer's	62.5					
0900			Ringer's	62.5	375				
1000			Ringer's	62.5		vomit	205		
1100	Juice	200	Ringer's	62.5					
1200			Ringer's	62.5	220				
1300			Ringer's	62.5					
1400	Water	150	Ringer's	62.5	265				
1500									
1600									
1700									
1800									
1900									
2000									
2100									
2200									
2300									
2400									
Totals		675		437.5	860		205		
Total Input		1112.5			**Total Output**		1065		

Fluid balance for time period = 1112.5 – 1065 = 47.5ml

Figure 8.2   Susan Stay's FBC

c. Fluid balance was covered in Chapter 4 (Fluid balance and maintenance) and you should refer back to it for revision if needed.

Fluid balance = Total input – Total output

Total input = 325 + 62.5 + 62.5 + 62.5 + 200 + 62.5 + 62.5 + 62.5 + 62.5 + 150 = 1112.5

The 200ml of water at 1600 is not included as this is later in time than was asked in this question.

Total output = 375 + 205 + 220 + 265 = 1065

The 135ml of urine at 1600 is not included as this is later in time than was asked in this question.

Therefore Susan has a fluid balance of:

1112.5 – 1065 = 47.5ml

Answer: 47.5ml fluid balance

d. Susan's IV of Lactated Ringer's Solution is due to be completed 16 hours after it was started. Since it was started at 8 a.m., which is 0800, you need to add 16 hours to this figure. This means the IV is scheduled to complete at midnight, which is 2400hrs.

Answer: Midnight or 2400hrs

e. The calculation of IV rates is covered in Chapter 6 (Calculating intravenous rates) and you should refer back to this for revision.

$$\text{IV rate} = \frac{\text{IV amount in ml} \times \text{giving set}}{\text{Hours} \times 60}$$

$$\text{IV rate} = \frac{1000 \times 20}{16 \times 60} = 20.8 \text{ drops/minute}$$

The cancelling down of fractions was covered in Chapter 2 (Essential numeracy requirements for nursing). This result must now be rounded as seen in Chapter 2; as the decimal is over half way the amount will be rounded up and you may wish to revise this chapter for both skills.

Answer: IV rate 21 drops/minute

f. Susan is prescribed 4 milligrams of apomorphine from a stock strength of 0.04g/ml. You are asked to calculate the correct dose to be given to Susan.

The calculation of drug dosages was covered in Chapter 5 and if needed you should refer to it for revision practice. You may also want to revise Chapter 3 (Quantity conversions for nurses) as one of the given amounts will need converting in this question.

0.04g/ml = 40mg/ml

Now to the actual dosage calculation.

Need = 4mg   **H**ave = 40mg   **S**tock = 1ml

$$\frac{N}{H} \times \frac{S}{1} = \text{The correct dose for the patient}$$

$$\frac{4}{40} \times \frac{1}{1} = 0.1\text{ml}$$

(Remember to put the unit of measure in your answer.)

The cancelling down of fractions was covered in Chapter 2 (Essential numeracy requirements for nursing) and you may wish to revise this chapter.

Answer: 0.1ml of apomorphine is the correct dose for Susan

g. Susan is to receive mitoxantrone injections that have been prescribed at $12mg/m^2$ for a body surface area (BSA) of $1.5m^2$.

Dosage of a patient using their BSA was covered in Chapter 7 (Calculations and children). Given Susan has a BSA of $1.5m^2$ and was prescribed 12 milligrams for each square metre, the calculation to find her required dose would be:

$$1.5 \times 12 = 18$$

The multiplication of numbers with decimals was covered in Chapter 2 (Essential numeracy requirements for nursing).

You now know Susan requires 18 milligrams of mitoxantrone and must calculate the amount to be drawn up.

The calculation of drug dosages was covered in Chapter 5 and if needed you should refer to it for revision practice. There is no requirement to convert any of the amounts in this calculation as both weights are in milligrams.

Need = 18mg **H**ave = 2mg **S**tock = 1ml

$$\frac{N}{H} \times \frac{S}{1} = \text{The correct dose for the patient}$$

$$\frac{18}{2} \times \frac{1}{1} = 9ml$$

Answer: 9ml of mitoxantrone is the correct dose

h. Susan's weight is 80 kilograms. The dosage prescribed 1.5mg/kg/day. The drug is available in Pre-Filled Syringes of strength 20mg, 40mg, 60mg, 80mg and 100mg and you are tasked to calculate how many injections and what strength Susan should be given daily so that she receives the correct amount of Clexane each day.

Dosage of a patient using their weight was covered in Chapter 7 (Calculations and children). Given Susan has a recorded weight of 80 kilograms and was prescribed 1.5 milligrams for each kilogram, the calculation to find her required dose would be:

$$80 \times 1.5 = 120mg$$

The multiplication of numbers was covered in Chapter 2 (Essential numeracy skills for nurses).

You now know Susan requires 120 milligrams of Clexane and must calculate how many injections she is to be given daily. Looking at the strength given for the Pre-Filled Syringes, 120mg is possible so that you will be able to give her 120mg in a combination.

Answer: To get 120mg you need a 100mg and a 20mg Pre-Filled Syringe or two 60mg Pre-Filled Syringes

Answers to the NMP tests

NMP Test 1

Q1 105 tablets

Q2 10 millilitres

Q3 625 milligrams

Q4 28 tablets

Q5 2.3 milligrams

NMP Test 2

Q1 35 tablets

Q2 12 millilitres

Q3 625 milligrams

Q4 21 tablets

Q5 1.875 milligrams

NMP Test 3

Q1 21 tablets

Q2 8 millilitres

Q3 775 milligrams

Q4 7 tablets

Q5 1.25 milligrams

NMP Test 4

Q1 42 tablets

Q2 3.2 millilitres

Q3 1375 milligrams

Q4 31.5 or $31\frac{1}{2}$ tablets

Q5 1.215 milligrams

NMP Test 5

Q1 42 tablets

Q2 4ml

Q3 172mcg

Q4 40 tablets

Q5 0.53mg *or* 0.530mg

Glossary

Dactinomycin: A highly toxic drug used in chemotherapy regimens for the treatment of renal cancer in children.

Drip chamber: The use of a drip chamber allows an estimate of the rate at which fluid is administered for an intravenous (IV) infusion.

Essential Skills Clusters: Skills and behaviours that students will need to demonstrate in order to prove achievement in specified competencies.

Fluid balance: The difference between fluid input and fluid output.

Fluid Balance Chart(s): Records a patient's hourly fluid intake and output over a specified time period.

Fluid intake: The amount of fluid a patient consumes via oral drinks, food, intravenous fluids or tube feeds.

Fluid output: The amount of fluid a patient excretes via urine, vomiting, tube drainage, diarrhoea, gastric secretions or wound drainage.

Giving set: A device used to break down the flow of each millilitre of fluid, from an IV infusion, into droplets.

Injection/Intravenous (IV) infusion: An injection is an infusion method of putting fluid into the body, usually with a hollow needle and a syringe which is pierced through the skin to force fluid into a vein or tissue.

Macrodrip: A chamber that converts each millilitre of fluid, from an IV infusion, into 15 or 20 drops.

Microdrip: A chamber that converts each millilitre of fluid, from an IV infusion, into 60 drops.

Neonate: A small child or baby.

Nephroblastoma: Tumour of the kidneys found mostly in children; also known as Wilms' Tumour.

Nomogram: A graphical calculating device, a two-dimensional diagram designed to allow the approximate graphical computation of a function, in this case the surface area of a human body.

Oncologist: A medical professional who practises oncology; oncology is a branch of medicine that deals with tumours (cancer).

Orally: By mouth (e.g. many drugs are taken orally).

Paediatrician: A doctor or consultant who deals with the medical care of infants, children and adolescents.

Plasma: Blood plasma is the yellow liquid component of blood, in which the blood cells in whole blood would normally be suspended.

Platelets: These are small, irregularly shaped anuclear cells (i.e. cells that do not have a nucleus containing DNA) which form clots in blood.

Prime number: A number which is exactly divisible by only 1 and itself.

Registrar: A medical doctor in the UK receiving advanced training in a specialist field.

Stock strength or dispensed dose: The amount of drug as kept in a specified strength in the pharmacy or on the ward in the medicine cabinet.

Strength required or prescribed strength: The amount of drug to be given to the patient.

Subcutaneous: An injection administered as a bolus into the subcutis, which is the layer of skin directly below the dermis and epidermis.

Ventricular arrhythmias: A condition in which there is abnormal activity in the heart.

Volumetric pump: A pump that is used to deliver rates of fluid intravenously at 5ml or more per hour.

Drug calculations

N is for **Need**; **H** is for **Have**; **S** is for the **stock volume**

Put them together and you get

$$\frac{N}{H} \times \frac{S}{1} = \text{The correct dose for the patient}$$

The ladder to Successful Nursing

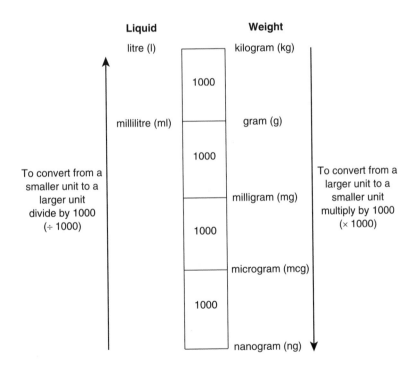

Liquid

Weight

litre (l)

kilogram (kg)

1000

millilitre (ml)

gram (g)

1000

To convert from a
smaller unit to a
larger unit
divide by 1000
(÷ 1000)

milligram (mg)

To convert from a
larger unit to a
smaller unit
multiply by 1000
(× 1000)

1000

microgram (mcg)

1000

nanogram (ng)

IV rate calculations

$$\frac{\text{Amount of IV in millilitres} \times \text{giving set}}{\text{Number of hours} \times 60} = \text{Number of drops per minute}$$

The ladder for height conversion

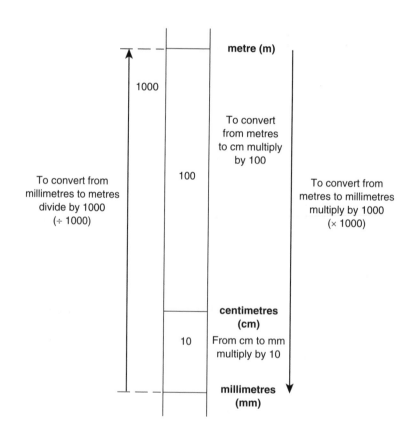

metre (m)

1000

To convert
from metres
to cm multiply
by 100

100

To convert from
millimetres to metres
divide by 1000
(÷ 1000)

To convert from
metres to millimetres
multiply by 1000
(× 1000)

**centimetres
(cm)**

10   From cm to mm
multiply by 10

**millimetres
(mm)**

Index